What Lies Behind the Smile

By Nicole Moneer

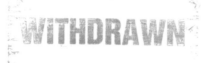

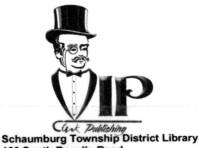

A smile can hide a lot of pain.
A smile may be all that is needed to work through the pain.
A smile may be the cure to rid your body of pain. - Unknown

"A smile on my face doesn't mean my life is perfect; it means I appreciate what I have and what God blessed me with." - Unknown

"It's easy to look at people and make quick judgments about them, their presents and their pasts, but you'd be amazed at the pain and tears a single smile hides. What a person shows to the world is only one tiny facet of the iceberg hidden from sight. And more often than not, it's lined with cracks and scars that go all the way to the foundation of their soul." - Sherrily Kenyon

To every person who reads this book, I thank you for taking the time to do so. I know that most all of you can relate to putting on a mask ... a smile, many times throughout your life to cover up your pain and your problems. We all do it.

Nicole Moneer

Contents

Chapter 1 - Intro

Today is Sunday April 12, 2012. I just inked a book deal with VIP Ink Publishing, L.L.C., to whom I am grateful, on March 10th 2012. March 10th also happens to be the day my mother passed away unexpectedly.

I dedicate my book to both my parents. I would not be where I am today without them both, especially my mom. I believe that if you think you can do something, you can. A lot of my success is due to my positive mindset and my mother's encouragement, support, and unconditional love. She was a constant presence throughout my entire life. I love this quote so much, and it's what my book and life are truly about:

> *"If you learn from your suffering and really come to understand the lesson you were taught you might be able to help someone else who is now in the phase you may have just completed. Maybe that's what it's all about after all." - Anonymous*

I hope you enjoy reading my life story. Some people might come to a different opinion of me after reading it, but this is why I am sharing it. Many think most peoples' lives are perfect, which is a farce. No one is perfect, so no one has room to judge anyone else, their decisions, or their lives. However, we are all guilty of judging one another. I share my story to show that I am not different from anyone else, and that you are not alone. I have encountered and overcome many hardships and struggles with different issues throughout my life. I have overcome so much and I continue to move forward. But I am not perfect! I am a sinner like everyone else. I have learned and am still learning, but most importantly, I have been able to take a look at myself and make the necessary life changes to better myself and move closer to God. In the end, isn't that what it's all about?

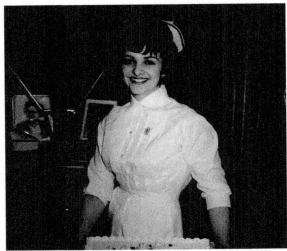

Mary Moneer in uniform during her time at Resurrection Hospital

My Parents

I was born November 29, 1972 in Oak Park, IL at West Suburban Hospital. My dad's name is Yusuf Moneer, and he was born February 13, 1939 in Pune, India. His family migrated to Pakistan after it became a country. He passed away June 9, 1996. I never met my paternal grandfather; I think he passed away before I was born. I did meet my paternal grandmother. She lived with us for a while during my high school and college years. My dad has one brother and two sisters. One of his brothers lived in Pakistan, and he passed away a few years ago. He has a sister, Kay, who lives in California, and his other sister is in a mental institution. My dad received his medical degree while living in Pakistan. He later practiced Hematology and Oncology in the USA. He came to the US in the mid-sixties sometime around 1965 and did his internship at Resurrection Hospital.

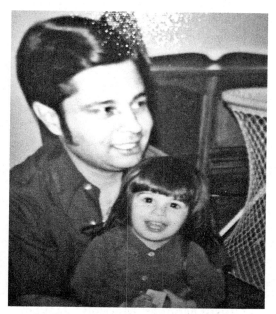

Nicole with Father, Yusuf Moneer

My mom, Mary Kottra, was born on December 19, 1942. Mary was born in Chicago to Julius and Rose Kottra. She was a nurse, and while working at Resurrection Hospital, she met my dad. My dad had great references from his school in Pakistan which led to him working at Resurrection. They were engaged in early 1966 and married on November 5, 1966. They started out in an apartment in Oak Park, IL, and my brother, who prefers to remain anonymous, was born August 12, 1967. Soon after, they bought a home close to my mom's parents and lived there for a few years. Then they moved to Western Springs, IL where my father opened a practice in an office with four other doctors. We lived in Western Springs until I was about four years old. I was born November 29, 1972. My mom named me after a soap opera star on *The Edge of Night*.

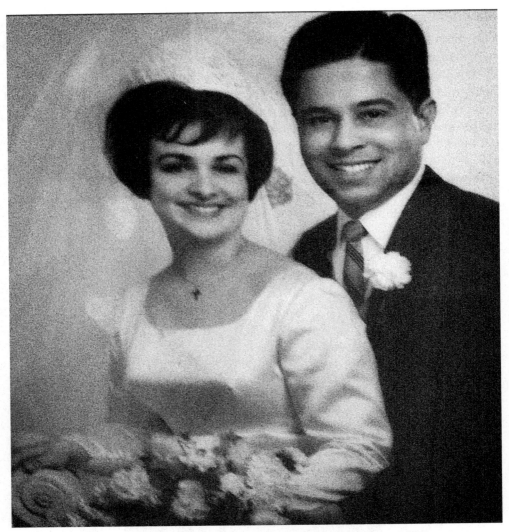

Mary and Yusuf Moneer, Married 5 November 1966

Since my brother prefers to remain anonymous, we shall call him "Brother Anonymous," so for the rest of the book we'll call him BA **:)**. He is my older brother and
was born in 1967. One of my earliest memories of BA was when my family was in
Seattle while he was going through all his testing. My brother was diagnosed with
leukemia, and in the '70s he only had a 10% chance of survival. He needed a bone
marrow transplant to save his life. Both of my parents were tested, and neither
was a match. I was tested and was found to be a perfect match. I remember being
in the halls at the hospital after the bone marrow transplant took place. My dad
was there with me, and I had a banana-split after the surgery. Some of the testing
they did back then was scary. I remember some of the skin testing, and it was painful.

My brother was the only one of the patients on his floor who survived; again, he had only a 10% chance of survival at that time. His doctor invented the bone marrow transplant and later won the Nobel Prize in Medicine. I remember my brother asking if he was going to die, and I remember my dad telling me "I hope not." We became friends with a family while temporarily living in Seattle, and I am still friends with them today through Facebook. Their daughter who was a cancer patient on my brother's floor did not survive. My brother is a miracle. It's incredibly ironic that I saved his life. I never thought that in my career I would also be saving

countless others with nutrition, exercise, and emotional support. We, as a family, travelled back to The Fred Hutchinson Cancer Research Center in Seattle every two years for about 10 years for BA's check-ups.

Brother Anonymous Childhood Memories

Nicole Janet Moneer was born on November 29, 1972. I was five years old and vaguely remember her arrival. I remember Mom coming home with my little sister in a blanket. Little did I know that that tiny baby would save my life about five years later. Of course, Nicky got all the attention and got away with everything. She was a feisty one. It wasn't too long before Mom, and the rest of us, started calling her "Picky Nicky" as she was fussy about everything from her toys to what she ate. She is still fussy about what she eats - for obvious reasons. I remember that she would call her food different names; bananas were called "mina." She had her own code language. Our father was a physician who often made rounds at the local hospital. Nicky would ask if Dad was at the "hopsickle." If she didn't get what she wanted, she would throw a tantrum. Dad would just laugh and let her get away with it, but not me. We will revisit this a bit later.

I remember one Christmas when Nicky was six and I was eleven. Aunt Beverly and Uncle Ron came by Christmas Eve in 1978 with their two older boys, but did not bring their little toddler, Jenny. Nicky opened their gift of dollhouse furniture and had a royal tantrum in front of everyone. I will never forget it because my dad would have kicked my ass if I would have done anything like that. She threw the furniture across the room at the Christmas tree and started shouting, "I don't want stupid furniture! I want Jenny!" Well, in hindsight, most coaches of athletes will tell you that this is the kind of "difficult" personality it takes to mold a champion.

As I said, my father was very strict and abusive with me physically and mentally throughout my childhood until my teen years when I was grounded for much of them. He was a medical resident at this time from 1967-1971. He immigrated to this country from Karachi, Pakistan in 1964 to begin his medical training in Chicago, IL where he met our mom who was working as a nurse. First, my father had a very short temper. Starting when I was two years old, he would smack me across the head, call me names like "idiot head" and swear at me. From that time on, being

4

around my father was like walking on eggshells or walking through a minefield. I never knew what was going to set him off and I was still too young to understand what was going on. At this time, Mom, Dad, and I lived just a mile or two from my maternal grandparents. Grandpa paid the down payment on the Caldwell house which may have caused some financial upheaval. Mom tried to protect me but did not say anything about the way Dad was mistreating me because our grandparents would have been very upset.

Nicky was not born until 1972 after we moved from Caldwell about 30 miles away to our new home in Western Springs, a suburb of Chicago. While we were in the Western Springs home, I may have been 6 or 7 and Nicky was 1 or 2, I was playing in the neighbor's yard with Matt and Mary Anne, neighborhood kids, and we had yoyos. I was yo-yoing and swinging it around, and it slipped and broke their garage window (it was a small, cheap plastic window). When I got home, I knew I was going to be in big trouble. I pleaded with Mr. Russo, "Please don't tell my Dad. I'll pay for it," but he did. So when I got home, I was beaten with the nozzle of a vacuum cleaner and then thrown down the stairs. My mom tried to stop him. Another incident happened when I was 5 or 6. I was playing with my friend, Michael. He was swinging on the horse swing set. He fell off the swing and started crying. My dad chased me around the house and I hid but after a while, when he found me, he threw me down the stairs.

I remember in the spring of my second grade in 1975, I kept crying to my dad, a physician specializing in hematology and oncology for adults, that I had severe bone pain in my right foot. My mom was an R.N. No one really understood what was going on with me until about six months later. Then, one Sunday in July 1975, just before my eighth birthday, my breathing became very heavy and labored. I felt like I was suffocating, like I couldn't get enough air with each breath. So my dad took me to Children's Memorial Hospital where they admitted me and performed a series of blood tests. Then Dr. Helen Maurer, the top pediatric hematologist in Chicago at the time, told me that my blood test was not normal and that she had to do a bone marrow aspiration test, whatever that was. I asked the nurse if it hurt. She said, "It feels like a little pinch." I will never forget that because she was full of it.

They make you lie on your stomach and nurses and doctors hold the patient down while the doctor injects Novocain to supposedly numb the skin and tissue over the tail bone. Then they take a large drill needle with another thinner needle inside the drill needle and drill a hole into the tail bone. Then the thinner needle sucks out the bone marrow inside the bone, which unequalizes the pressure inside the bone causing more pain. Although they give you Novocain, they cannot numb the bone tissue; only the flesh above the bone gets numb. It is normally a ten minute procedure. Little did I know that I would have to endure many of these bone marrow aspiration tests over the next four years. These bone marrow tests were by far the worst part of my childhood; even worse than the abuse from my father. My dad and Dr. Maurer told me I had leukemia. I was only eight years old but I knew that leukemia was a form of cancer, and that people died from it because my dad always talked about his leukemia patients with my mom. I asked Dad if I was going to die. He said he hoped not, but he didn't know.

That began the intense regime of chemotherapy and radiation treatments for eight weeks, which was another unpleasant part of my childhood. I lost my hair and had to wear a wig in third grade in addition to enduring repeated bone marrow tests. I had hundreds of blood tests, which didn't bother me in the least bit as I was just happy it was not a bone marrow test or a spinal tap. A few months later, I got the shingles virus because I was immune-compromised from the chemo treatments. This was another nasty part of childhood, as shingles is an ugly series of very painful warts and cysts with fluid in them. I was laid up at home for two weeks on codeine medications at the age of eight. The meds only slightly took the edge off the pain but did not relieve the blemishes. It took another three months for the blemishes and scars to heal up. About six months later, my hair grew back and things started to return to normal.

On April 15th 1977, at the age of 9, I was told that my blood tests were abnormal again, so they were taking me to the hospital for a bone marrow test and a spinal tap. On this day, I ran down the fire escape to avoid the bone marrow test. They eventually caught up with me. My dad and seven doctors and nurses took me to the examination room where they held me down. They had to do the bone marrow test six times to get a proper sample from me and then they had to do a spinal tap four times to get the fluid sample. Then they told me I had relapsed; the leukemia, ALL (acute lymphocytic leukemia), had resurfaced its ugly head.

My dad and mom told me that after the first relapse the leukemia would inevitably take my life in one to three years' time unless I went up for a bone marrow transplant. But first they had tried to get me into a second remission before going up for the transplant, since the chances of survival are greatly increased for patients who are in remission. So there I went for another round of intense chemo and radiation. They did get me back into remission for the transplant. In the meantime, they tested my family members to see if anybody was a good HLA tissue type match for me; this goes way beyond merely having matching blood types. At that time, it was not possible to have a donor who was not related to the patient in his or her immediate family. Many patients had up to six siblings and none of them matched, but fortunately for me, my sister, Nicole, was a perfect tissue match as if she were an identical twin. She was only four years old at the time, and I was nine going on ten.

Dr. E. Donnall Thomas at the Fred Hutchinson Cancer Research Center, the inventor of the bone marrow transplant procedure, was the lead physician on my medical team of top cancer researchers. He was the first physician to be awarded the

Nobel Prize for his clinical work in inventing and perfecting the bone marrow transplant procedure in 1992. Unfortunately, he recently passed away in 2012 in his nineties, but his legacy lives on. My mom, dad, and doctors told me I had a 10% chance of making it through the transplant because of the rigorous supra-lethal total body radiation and intense chemo required to kill every blood and bone marrow cell in my body to make way for the new donor marrow to come from Nicole. I remember Dr. Thomas administered the entire dose of 1000 rads of total body radiation in 3 hours' time (now they give it over 5 days- hyperfractionated dosing). I went in a normal happy kid in remission and came out a very sick prune. I lost my hair again very soon afterward. On that same day, August 9, 1977, the doctors put 4 year-old Nicole to sleep and aspirated large quantities of bone marrow from her hips and tail bones. I was grateful for the donation, of course, but I was a bit jealous only because she at least got general anesthesia for her bone marrow harvesting, and I never got the luxury of being put to sleep. But this was because they were taking larger quantities of bone marrow at one time from Nicole. She was a bit sore for the next couple of days, but recovered quickly.

Bone marrow is like blood; it is the most rapidly replicating tissue in the body. They put Nicole's bone marrow in an I.V. machine and slowly administered it to me. They don't know exactly how, but bone marrow finds its way to the bone marrow cavities when injected intravenously. I turned 10 three days later on August 12, 1977. I remember trying to eat my mom's spaghetti, but I could not tolerate or even taste it. The chemo and radiation had altered my taste buds. I was constantly vomiting several times a day as well. They also had to sterilize my food and drink because I had to keep everything sterile, and I mean everything, outside as well as inside my body.

Now comes the real fun. I had to remain in a sterile plastic bubble for fifty days while my immune system recovered enough to live outside it. In the meantime, I had weekly spinal taps and bone marrow tests. Not fun. I hated these tests. I knew that I would get out of there one way or the other. Either the Lord Jesus would take me and spare me of this, or he would heal me and I would recover. After a long 49 days, I put my sterile clothes and mask on, ran out of my bubble after midnight on day 49 and greeted the nurses, doctors, and cooks. They were really pissed at me but I could not figure out why. I protested, "It's Day 50!!" They told me to get back in. I got out the next day but strangely they told me I could go back home to Chicago instead of staying at a nearby apartment complex for another 50 days as required for most patients who make it past the 50th day.

A few years later, I found out that the doctors took my bone marrow and told my parents I had relapsed. The slide showed bone marrow cells that looked like cancerous cells. A few months later, my dad took another bone marrow sample and showed it to Dr. Maurer, and the cancer was gone. It turned out that my male bone marrow cells were immature and had not been completely killed off and mixed with my sister's bone marrow, which are identifiable as female bone marrow cells. Normally, when the host (cancer patient's) cells come back, they previously thought that always meant that the cancer had come back. In my case, however, it was a case of mistaken identity, thank the Lord! My cells did come back, but they were immature and thus mistaken for cancer cells.

The next phase of the recovery wasn't so bad. I got to stay home from school for nine months, the entire academic year of my fifth grade. I had to stay home from school and away from other crowded places until my immune system fully recovered. I walked around the block with my mom and had a tutor for a couple of hours a day. I really accomplished nothing of substance in fifth grade, but was passed right on to sixth grade and even earned math honors awards. I had been listening to music while I was in the bubble; groups like Aerosmith and Heart. I decided I really wanted to play electric guitar when I got home, and I did.

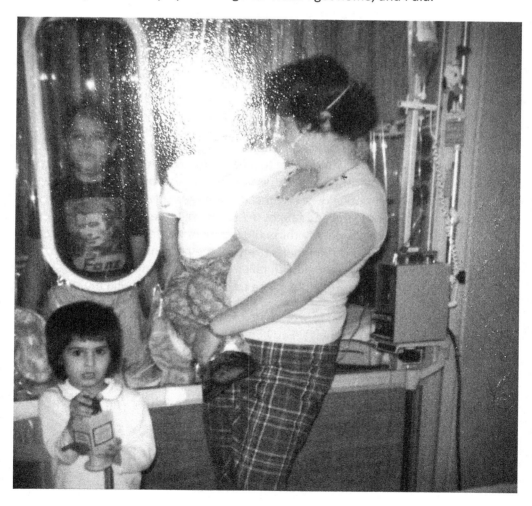

In the Bubble; Seattle, Washington

Chapter 2 - My Younger Years

"From birth to death we are never pain-free. Even the greatest people in the world and in the Bible have made the gravest mistakes. You're gonna go through the ringer, so hang on tight. We are set free in our pain. We are rescued in our pain. When we crash and burn, we see things and people in different and refreshing ways." - Tony Evans

When I was younger, around age five or six, my father left home a few times. He told me that the only reason he stayed with my mom at our house was because of me. In 1981, he received a letter from the Department of Child and Family Services. My mom had reported him and his abuse so if he physically abused my brother or me again, he would go to jail.

At age four, I began taking ballet tap and jazz at a dance studio in our area. I later continued with high school and college Poms. When children are involved in competition, hobbies, or teams at a young age, it greatly benefits them in their adult years. It teaches them how to work with other people, and how to bond and build friendships. They learn early on that it's not about them, but rather about the group. It also gives them self-confidence, it teaches them how to cope with pressure later on in life and more importantly, it keeps them active and healthy. I took ballet tap and jazz for thirteen years. My mom attended my dance recitals but my dad rarely did. My mom was always proud of me and taking tons of photos up until the day she died. I really loved my first teacher, too; Priscilla Santi was the best. She was very loving and caring, and this is very important for a teacher. The best part of dance and competing over the decades has been my coaches. I appreciate how they have mentored me and taught me so much, none of which I could ever have learned from a textbook. My thirty plus years of dance and being on stage gave me a backbone; a thick skin to deal with all the hardships life has thrown at me. I learned early on how to deal with failure and became more perseverant. Looking back now, being enrolled in dance class really helped build my self-esteem.

My parents always taught me to work hard for things. My mom and dad never allowed me to get away with things. Early on, I knew the meaning of "no." My parents, especially my father, were always hard on me, along with my coaches and bosses. This created my mindset of "I can and I will," pushing ahead and through, knocking down doors, and so on. Most people don't like to hear "no"; I heard "no" a lot from my dad, from jobs, and throughout my life. All those "no's" taught me to work harder and to never give up.

Priscilla Santi - My First Dance Teacher

Nicole was with me from the ages of 4-12; at the time we had the dance review. It was pretty early on, our third year in business, when she was with me. I was in business for 20 years. She was very focused, even as a young child, and she stayed with it the whole time. Most don't stay with dance, and this has a big impact on them. They move from taking one class to taking four classes. This is a lot for a 12 year old to be doing; staying focused was noticeable in her. She could stay focused whether she was in ballet, tap or jazz class. Now if you're good in dance, you're good in sports, so then you might be going in ten different directions. The ability to stay focused tells you a lot about a person at an early age. Not only that, but Nicole could dance well, too.

When you're little and you take dance and love it, it opens up a whole new world. It helps in your ability to speak in front of a lot of people, and work well with others, too. We had really good teachers and this helped greatly. At the time Nicole was coming to my studio, we had one of the first tap dancers in Chicago. He was in WWII, and then he came to our school. His way of teaching was amazing. Mr. Sutton has passed, but his daughter still teaches.

We were just getting off the ground at the time, and I remember Nicole was so cute! She had little dark features and at that age, all the children are all about the same height. When they come in at 4, they like to be with a friend and they like to couple up. When they look into the mirror, some kids will do jazz and see themselves in that venue. When she looked in the mirror, Nicole was more ballet; she was more on her tip-toes. She wanted to jump and stuff like that.

Like I said, Nicole was very focused, more than the other children. I was just learning how to teach at the same time she was learning how to dance. There would be 20 children in a class, and while I had good students--they all were great--I would put her at the start of the line, because the other kids could watch her and see what they needed to do, too. She never cried or pouted, she would always listen, and she was a very good student.

It was still new to everyone; I did not know that she could have a career in this. Once they got into that first year of high school, it was then that something might have shown. When looking back, I was surprised to see how many of the girls did go into modeling. Nicole had a lot of music talent within her; I only knew her as a little kid; however, I could tell she was

rhythmic. She could hear the music, and how to add the right steps to the beats, and so forth. For a little kid that is a huge task to be able to do.

I think it's exciting to see where she is now and I think her life is just starting. She has become a beautiful women.

Grade School

During my Catholic grade school years, I was teased and bullied, mainly in sixth grade but also a little in second grade. I am positive this was a huge influence on many aspects of my life today.

From Don't Wait Project by Lisa Bradshaw:

Did you know?
1 out of 4 teens are bullied.
9 out of 10 students experience harassment at school or online.
As many as 160,000 students stay home on any given day because they're afraid of being bullied.
1 in 5 kids admits to being bullied or doing some "bullying."
43% fear of being harassed in the bathroom at school.
282,000 students are physically attacked in secondary schools each month.
More youth violence occurs on school grounds than on the way to school.
(www.dontwaitproject.org)

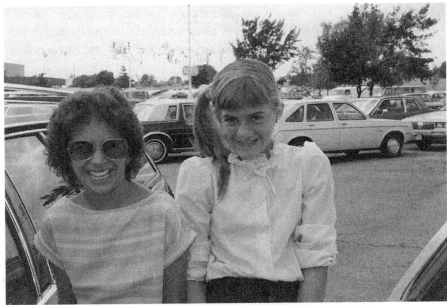

Nicole Moneer and friend, 1983 (6th Grade)

I remember a few things about being teased during my grade school days (sixth and seventh grades) on the bus and from neighborhood kids. I was bullied about how I looked. Kids are mean. My mom had no clue how to do hair; she never did her own hair. I never wore braids, pony-tails, curls, or anything cute and girly in my younger years. My mom took me to The Pomp Room where she had her hair done. Over the years, I had a bowl haircut, a mullet, and lastly a super curly perm. Are you laughing yet? It's OK, you can. My mom wore prescription eyeglasses that tinted in the sun and she bought me the same since I needed a prescription starting in sixth grade. At recess, I was made fun of since my glasses changed when I went outside in daylight. Can you picture these? When outside at recess, this was so not cool. I was also often made fun of because the shoes my mother had bought for me were from Nordstrom. Penny Loafers, Top Siders, and flats with bobby socks were "in" but I had Famolares, a super ugly brown orthopedic looking shoe. In the early eighties, these types of wedges were not in; now they are. I guess I was ahead of the trend, ha! Once I entered seventh grade though, I became sort of cool because I was the first to wear Guess jeans. I was making money working for my mom's craft show business, so I started to buy myself shoes and clothes, and I even learned how to style my own hair. I did have a small crush on someone but he never saw me in the same way, at least not until high school. We dated in high school briefly--only for two weeks. This person was my first rejection. It is funny how a few years after grade school when my look changed, he took an interest in me. Maybe the fashionista in me had come out from this teasing thing. For those of you who have been teased or bullied in grade school, high school, or even as an adult, I know you can relate, and on a positive note, you may even agree that it forced you to do things you may not otherwise have done. It's ironic that my mom saved some of my grade school report cards. I received A's and B's mainly, but C's in PE! Can you believe it? At this point, I've been a holistic health and fitness professional for 16 plus years. Who would have guessed?

When my brother was in eighth grade, I was about eight years old. I do not remember all of the details, but my father was upset with my brother. I recall my dad telling my brother that he wished my brother was dead. My brother then ran away from home. I remember my mom and me driving all over the place looking for him. We found him at the Oasis on the toll way, which was not too far from where we lived at the time. Another time, we were at my grandparent's house. My brother found their liquor cabinet and drank so much that he overdosed and had to have his stomach pumped. This was my first experience with alcohol. I watched my brother slumped naked in the bath tub, slurring his words; he couldn't move. He had blacked out. My mom called my Uncle Jerry to lift him up out of the bath tub, so they could take him to the ER. My Uncle Jerry has done a lot for my mom and our family over the years, especially things my mother could not count on my father to do. My mom could not call my dad for fear of what he would do, plus, he was the reason my brother overdosed. Following this episode, my BA was sent to rehab and counseling for a period of time. You'll see later how alcohol kept coming into my life through others, and how sensitive I am to it.

Sophomore year of high school, I was nominated for Pom Squad Captain and the squad and I went to summer camp. I remember that as a captain, at age 15, I took that responsibility as a way to boss people around because I thought I was better than they were. I also learned at age 15 that pushing others around is not what a leadership role is at all. I thought I was the best dancer too and even spoke down to some of the girls. Our squad did not do well at camp that year, mainly because of my poor leadership. When you have a good leader, you have a good team, but when you have a bad leader, you have a bad team. When appointed to lead others, you work for your people; it's not about you, it's about them.

At 15 going on 16, my dad had received my report card, which was not to his liking. He told me I could no longer be on the pom squad. I was devastated! This lasted for about a week, thank you God. Then my dad allowed me to go back on the team. Senior year, I was co-captain of Varsity Poms. That year, we did better as a squad; we also had a lot of practices at my house. There were six of us choreographing our summer camp routine. We ended up winning as a squad, and many won individual ribbons too for individual competitions. Since Jeannine (the captain) and I did so well at NCA camp, we were selected to fly to New York and perform in the 1989 Macy's Thanksgiving Day Parade. This was a great accomplishment for us both at such a young age. I even continued in college as a wrestling cheerleader and a pom squad member as well.

Thinking back to sophomore year of high school, my PE teacher was one of my dad's patients. Many people from our area trusted my dad as their primary care physician. Since my dad was well-known in the area, I had to be on my best behavior. Well, in PE class, I often talked to one guy. The teacher never said a word to me; he just wrote a letter to my dad stating that all I did in gym class was talk. My dad was so angry, he grounded me for the entire Christmas break, but compared to my BA, my punishment was nothing. My dad would ground him for a year at a time. Being the first child, he took most of the heat. Ironically, I got in trouble in high school PE and during my grade school years received bad grades, but now look at what I do for a living today!

My dad emotionally, verbally, and physically abused my brother and me. During my sophomore year of high school in the summer, I worked the Western Open. The last night of the event, my girlfriend and I lied to our parents. We told them we were attending a party after work at "so and so's" house, and that Michael Jordan, along with other celebrities, would be there. We ended up at another party, and were drinking and smoking pot. I was supposed to come home at midnight but instead, I made it home at 2 am. My dad had already called my girlfriend's mom. They were both driving around looking for us. When I got home, my dad grabbed me by my hair and slammed my head onto the concrete step. He yelled at me and grounded me for the rest of that summer. I had a little scrape and was bleeding some, but nothing that required a visit to the hospital.

I babysat the children of a good family friend during my high school summers. These people were always very supportive of me. When I was awarded MVP of Poms for my senior year of high school, my mom called them to let them know about my award and the event. They came to that event but my dad did not. I can't remember why he didn't come; I was 16 at the time. The Hanna family has always been there for me and still are to this day; thank you! They even attended my Lu-vabulls debut party for the Chicago Bulls. My dad did not attend that either, but he wasn't speaking to me at the time.

My father was not in my life much, at least not for important events. He was pretty strict with me regarding dating in high school. He was very hard on my brother though. Not only would BA be grounded for a year at a time, my dad sent him to military high school for two years. My brother was an A student, which didn't matter since he drank alcohol and smoked weed in his high school years. I admit, I often tattled on him when doing either. In high school I got busted for smoking cigarettes a few times by my dad, but nothing to the extent of the trouble my brother would get into. I was never busted for drinking alcohol or smoking weed. However, I was a typical sassy, snotty teenage girl. When we shopped for back-to-school clothes, my dad would either take them back or threaten to take them back if I sassed back to him or my mom. My dad never sat down and talked with my brother and me to explain what we did wrong. He just yelled at us or punished us. When I look at some of my clients, they sit down with their children, talk to them, explain right from wrong, and even ask their feelings. It is so important to connect and listen to your children versus just punishing them and not allowing them to speak. Let them be heard and explain right from wrong to them. My former client and now close friend, Maureen B., is awesome. She has excellent communication with her daughter. At 10, her daughter is happy, outgoing, and very well behaved.

After high school, I attended college. I received my BS degree in Fashion Merchandising from Iowa State University. I do like to be well put together from head to toe. Who doesn't? Well, I'm sure there are many of you out there to whom that may not be of any importance. When I rushed at Iowa State, I did it with a high school best friend during our sophomore year. I got accepted in to the Alpha Chi Omega house, but she did not get accepted in to any house. I know this hurt her. We lived together for about two semesters but when I moved into my sorority, she moved off campus. We did not see each other as often after that since we were both busy with other activities and lived apart.

During rush my sophomore year while at the Chi-Omega house, I encountered a girl who was a Chi-O, but two years older than I was, and who had lived down the street from me back home in Chicago. When I was six years old, the both of us were playing at a neighbor's house, and this girl who was a Chi-O was there as well.

I accidentally broke the cover of their record player. I was scared, so I ran home; I didn't know what to do. The next time I was at their home playing with her and the other girls, they were really mean to me. They kept picking on me, saying I had lice. I ran home crying. I was only six, and they were about eight. I did not have lice, and we never spoke again. Back to college and the Chi-Omega house, I sat down and talked to one of the girls; this was my second visit back at their house. The girls at every other house had been very nice to me. Well, this girl was pretty mean to me; she did not talk to me the entire time I was at their house. When girls rushed, at least 20 years ago when I did, the candidate would be with one girl and just with her the entire time while at the house, you know, to get to know each other to see if the candidates were a good fit. As it turns out, the mean girl from the neighborhood where I grew up had told my contact to ignore me during rush. An inside source, another Chi-Omega and a very good friend still to this day, confirmed this. This girl was still trying to get back at me even after all those years for the record player, or maybe she just thrived on being mean to other girls. Regardless, mean girls and mean people suck.

In college, my grades were not the best. I partied three days a week, and my GPA showed it too. In my freshman year, my dad told me to shape up or ship out. I slowly shaped up. However, I treated my body like a trash can, and it definitely spoke back to me. It took years before I listened and finally understood what my body was trying to tell me.

Chapter 3 - My Health History

"The Food you eat can be either the safest and most powerful form of medicine or the slowest form of poison." - Ann Wigmore

I was born sick. During my first three weeks of life, I had an upper respiratory infection, then four months later I came down with a fever. I received several immunizations at birth, and up until college: Measles, Rubella, Polio, Tetanus, Mumps, and Tuberculin in the '70s, '80s and 1990 when I graduated high school and entered college. In my teenage years, I became super ill when I was a sophomore in high school on spring break. I was in New York City visiting my Auntie Barbra. I remember sleeping upright on her sofa for most of the week since I had a hacking cough. My dad, being a doctor, was on the phone telling her what to give me; feed me this, go to the pharmacy and get her this, but nothing worked. Every year around spring time I would get sick like this. I would also have a hard time breathing and would get watery eyes! Many years later we found out I had an allergy to cats; my Auntie Barbara had three cats. I also was allergic to ragweed pollen, mold, and dust.

My menstrual cycle was always very hard on me during my high school years. I would often be in the nurse's office with a heating pad trying to get relief because the maximum amount of Advil wouldn't cut it. Later on in my thirties, when I made consistent dietary changes and added in certain supplements, I finally started to get relief from PMS. Senior year of high school I broke out with acne, but before this I had flawless skin. I did not need to wear makeup or anything. Of course, with my dad being a doctor, I had a referral for a top dermatologist. I was prescribed different antibiotics for my skin which kill the bad bacteria in the gut, but also kill the good/ friendly bacteria, too. This also creates a door to get sick more often, as friendly flora help fight off infections and so forth. I would stay on a prescription drug for X amount of time until it didn't work anymore, then my script would change to another drug. When I went off to Iowa State in 1990, my dad gave me a box of medicine "just in case" I got sick; "box" as in one of those large plastic bins you buy at Target with a snap close lid.

I was a typical college kid. I ate junk food late at night, drank a lot of beer and smoked cigarettes on weekends when drinking, or weeknights when up late studying. I rarely ate vegetables, proteins, fruits or healthy fats. I ate a lot of "dead" food. I was about 98 lbs. when I got out of high school; I looked "healthy" on the outside. I did enroll in college PE because I did not want to gain weight, aka the freshmen 15. I still did pack weight on in my second year of college from the abuse I put my body through from my poor food choices. It's funny, I weigh the same now as I did in college. In college I was a size six and while that is not big, it was for my body frame. The fat ratio of my body was 18-20% whereas now, at age 40, I am a size zero, weighing anywhere from 116-120 lbs., and my body fat ratio is around

12%. I have maintained this over the years since my eating habits are now a life-style and I've gained more lean muscle mass from weight training.

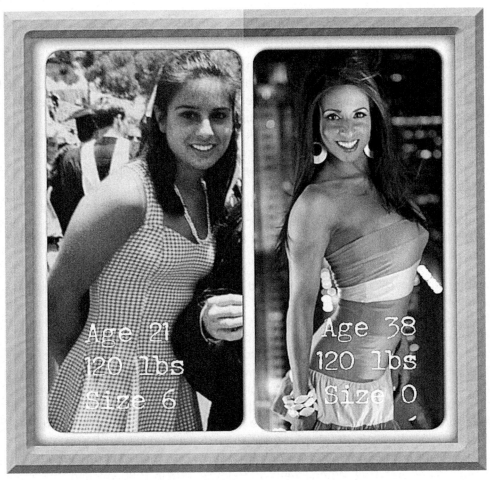

Age 21, 120 lbs, Size6,   vs.   Age 38, 120lbs, Size 0

In college I was sick often. I even had an abnormal pap smear when I was 20. I had to have surgery to remove pre-cancerous cells. My integrative doctor explained that if my pH balance is thrown off (as in being highly acidic), it can create problems throughout the body. I don't have any of the problems now like I did back when I was younger in my teens and twenties. I also am not on any prescription drugs and I don't eat a ton of highly acid "dead foods" like I did twenty years ago.

I was taking a lot of medicine that I did not need. I was not in a life threatening situation where I needed to take them. The foods I was eating were not helping either. In college, I had a lot of gastrointestinal stress, and I did not put two and two together until later in my thirties under the care of my integrative doctor. I could never drink (store bought) milk or eat yogurt from childhood up to my adult years. At 40 I tried raw milk and raw yogurt from a local farm for the first time, and I had no gastrointestinal problems. Did you know that pasteurized dairy creates inflammation in the body, as well as mucus, and most people are allergic and lactose-intolerant? Raw dairy is a much better choice and can be bought at a local farm. It's better because it contains all the good stuff that we need, like enzymes and antibodies that pasteurization kills. Raw dairy isn't plugged with hormones and antibiotics, which is what you get with store bought dairy. It's loaded with beneficial bacteria, enzymes and fat soluble vitamins.

I did not eat healthy when I was a kid. Neither did my parents. But I was active when I was a kid, with dance classes and Pom practice throughout high school and college. I was not doing resistance training; just cardio with all my dancing and performing. I was skinny fat! I looked healthy on the outside yet I was dying on the inside. So many people look and feel this way and live with it, not realizing that the power to turn their health around is in their own hands.

In college I had an ovarian cyst that ruptured. It was my freshmen year; I was 17 and we had a snow day. I remember being on the phone with my dad, crying in the hallway of my dorm because I was in so much pain. I had a roommate, and I did not want to wake her up, so I was out in the hall on the phone with my dad in the middle of the night. He asked all these questions, and then he told me I needed to get to the hospital. The ambulance came and got me on this snowy day. I sat in the ER for about five hours in major pain waiting for the doctor to arrive to examine me, under no pain killers whatsoever. They ruled out appendicitis and kidney stones and I was diagnosed with a ruptured ovarian cyst. It was very painful. Any of you ladies who have experienced this feel my pain, I am sure. I spent a few days in the hospital, and I missed the AC/DC concert with my best friend from high school.

I often went home from college for the holidays, summer break, and a few weekends throughout the year. When I did, I would go to my mom's place of employment for my allergy shots; she was an R.N. I did some allergy testing, a scratch test to be exact which is not as accurate as a blood/ food sensitivity test. It revealed what I was allergic to, foods included: dust, mold, pollen, and ragweed to name a few, but after seven years of being shot up with who knows what toxic chemicals, I was not getting any relief. My mom would even give me shots at home during non-office hours, since I couldn't always get in during their office hours. I was also on 2-3 inhalers for, well, almost two decades. During Christmas break freshmen year, I got super sick. I had to go back and cheer for wrestling meets during the holidays though.

When I went back to cheer, I took a train. I stayed with my girlfriend at her parents' home in Des Moines. People were allowed to smoke on the train at that time. Even though I smoked in high school and college socially, I could not tolerate being enclosed in the second hand smoke on the train. I could not smoke every day either; it was just too much. I smoked if I was up late studying or drinking on weekends. When I was enclosed in this smoke box train car, it was horrible. By the time I arrived in Des Moines, I was dying. I'd had about two hours of sleep that night since my friend had three cats, which I was allergic to at the time. I spent most of the night awake coughing and struggling to breathe. On the way to cheer for the first meet over holiday break, she took me to "student death" first. That was what we called Student Health in college. I hyperventilated in a paper bag all the way to "student death", which was about a thirty minute car ride. The doctor's orders: no cheering during the holiday break, and I was prescribed Prednisone and an inhaler, so I just watched the meets in the arena while sick and trying to recover.

At the beginning of my senior year of college, I went to the Registered Dietician per pep council directive. Each of us on the pom squad was required to do so. They want you to look the part and, of course, to be healthy. Some of the cheerleaders and even pom squad members struggled with eating disorders. I have never struggled with any eating disorder. They told me to cut out beef, cheese, and salad dressing. In college, I ate cheese pizza, cheesy beefs, and had Ranch dressing often. My family ate a lot of processed salad dressings too, like French and Thousand Island. Bad food choices begin in the home. My parents, a doctor and a nurse, taught me nothing about proper nutrition, yet so many people today follow their doctors' advice on how to eat. Today, I cannot imagine putting those processed dressings on my salads. I just add oil, vinegar, lemon or lime juices and apple cider vinegar to leafy greens with sea salt. YUM! I can't imagine ever going back. After removing the heavy salad dressings and cheese, I did slim down quite a bit and started to lose some of that freshman 15 body fat I had packed on.

During the tail end of my senior year when I was 21, I went into a bar full of smoke, and I could not breathe, so I left. I didn't pick up another cigarette again from that day forward until I met my husband at age 26. My eating habits did change, and I started to eat cleaner than before but nowhere near the level I am at today. No matter where you are on your health and fitness journey, know that you need to grow patience and take baby steps, and nutrition continually evolves.

After college I still was not eating 100% healthy, but I definitely wasn't drinking alcohol as much. I was going to the restroom a lot at work though because my GI distress was getting worse. I did not understand what it was. Certain foods would trigger it; I found out later on that it was IBS (irritable bowel syndrome). For those of you with this same problem, I know you can relate. When away from home, all I would focus on was where the bathroom was located.

Irritable bowel syndrome (IBS) is the most common functional gastrointestinal (GI) disorder with worldwide prevalence rates ranging from 9–23% and U.S rates generally in the area of 10–15%.

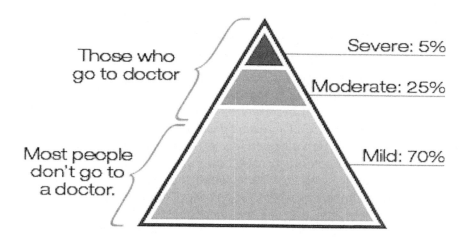

Those who go to doctor

Severe: 5%

Moderate: 25%

Most people don't go to a doctor.

Mild: 70%

Most people with IBS have mild symptoms. Many people don't recognize IBS symptoms. Yet, IBS is one of the most common disorders seen by physicians. Not all individuals with IBS symptoms seek medical care for their symptoms.

Nevertheless, there are between 2.4 and 3.5 million annual physician visits for IBS in the United States alone. IBS is the most common disorder diagnosed by gastroenterologists (doctors who specialize in digestive diseases or disorders) and accounts for up to 12% of total visits to primary care providers.

The cost to society in terms of direct medical expenses and indirect costs associated with loss of productivity and work absenteeism is considerable – estimates range from $21 billion or more annually.

A significant proportion – 35% to 40% – of individuals who report IBS in the community are male. Approximately 60% to 65% of individuals who report IBS in the community are female.

There is a suspected link between small intestine bacterial overgrowth (SIBO) and irritable bowel syndrome (IBS) because the two produce very similar symptoms. There is no test to confirm the existence of Irritable Bowel Syndrome, meaning it has always been difficult to diagnose. The elimination of other possibilities such as inflammation, infections, and cancer are typically how the diagnosis is achieved.

A hydrogen breath test is typically used to diagnose SIBO. This test often gives positive results for patients thought to have IBS. The ability of the patient to function normally in society is reduced drastically by both irritable bowel syndrome and small intestine bacterial overgrowth. Abnormal bowel habits such as alternating between extreme instances of constipation and diarrhea characterize irritable bowel syndrome. There is typically no drastic intervention since irritable bowel syndrome is not a life threatening condition. The importance of stress on overall health has become more prominent in recent years bringing this under question. Major health problems can result even though IBS is not a life threatening condition. There is often a fear of traveling long distances or eating in public places had by those suffering from IBS. Those suffering from the condition have a reduced quality of life resulting from the social embarrassment associated with major symptoms such as extreme gas and flatulence.

A number of doctors are starting to treat IBS patients without confirming SIBO's existence since the treatment of SIBO is often effective at the reduction of IBS symptoms. Oral antibiotics or probiotics are the most common treatments for small intestine bacterial overgrowth. Probiotics are beneficial bacteria that effectively compete with harmful bacteria found in the small intestines.

The overuse of antibiotics is the most controversial issue when it comes to the link between IBS and SIBO. An abnormality in the muscle tissue surrounding the intestines is what causes SIBO and probably IBS. The gas formation in IBS and bacterial overgrowth in SIBO is a result of the muscles being unable to move material effectively through the intestines which is the major cause of both SIBO and IBS. Oral antibiotics treat the secondary problem and not the actual cause. Oral antibiotics have to be given on a regular if not continual basis as a result in order to relieve symptoms.

A simple stool test can confirm enzyme and HCl deficiencies, along with bacterial and fungal imbalances which throw your digestion completely off-track. I discuss this later.

My poor gut was doomed from day 1 of life being plugged with drugs and not being breastfed. Pharmaceutical stress from the ongoing use of antac-ids, antibiotics, chemotherapy drugs and steroids can interfere with gut ecology adversely affecting digestion

I wanted to include this list of prescription drugs I was on to show the correlation between these drugs and my suffering health. I received allergy shots weekly for 7+ years for Mold, Dust Mite, Tree, Grass, Pollen, Ragweed, Dog, and Cat.

Flonase
Pulmicort
Azmacort
Albuterol
Allegra
Zyrtec
Intal
Nasacort
Hismanal
Violin/Clarithromycin
Z pak- Zithromax
Ceclor
Nordette and Ortho-Tri-Cyclen Birth Control from age 23-33 (I have been off birth control since 2006. Did you know that contraceptive pills have a devastating effect on the beneficial/good bacteria of the gut?)
Serafin for PMS
Diuretic Triamterene for PMS bloating

I stopped taking all of these drugs in 2006! I then started making better food choices and taking supplements under the care of my integrative doctor. My health has gotten better every day since. I do not get sick anymore with sinus in-fections, horrible PMS, chronic fatigue, asthma attacks or digestive problems, nor do I have the allergies listed above. I don't even use an inhaler anymore. All the chronic symptoms and conditions I had no longer exist. It took me months to heal my gut and a decade later I still make sure I put healing foods in my body.

After I graduated college, I was dating Life Lesson 3 (LL3), I am calling all past romances "Life Lessons", and working at Nordstrom when I felt excruciating pain on the left side of my abdomen. It hurt so much that I was doubled over in pain, I could not move and was rushed to the hospital. LL3 was there at the hospital with me. They had to rule out various diagnoses using the same steps as before, but once again, it was a ruptured ovarian cyst. This was the first time I had to have a catheter put in and the nurse then ripped it out of me. I don't ever want another catheter put in me again. It hurt like a MOFO! It's times like those that remind me of the importance of health and self-care. I was in the hospital overnight. I was still depressed due to my dad's recent unexpected death in June of 1996 and I was scared being in the hospital without him to care for me. I always knew I was in good hands with him; anytime I was sick, he always took care of me. Or was it just that he was always there to comfort me when sick, especially since he wasn't in my life much otherwise? This was very traumatic for me to be in the hospital without him. Since I was in the ER and hospital overnight, I missed my flight to Cancun. I planned a trip to travel during wintertime for vacation. In the meantime, my dad's best friend and partner in practice came in to take care of me, which is what I wanted. He had prescribed the birth control pill. He said this would help so I wouldn't ovulate. This happened again about two years later even while I was on the pill. I was rushed to the ER for a ruptured ovarian cyst three times in seven years. I have not had this happen since. My health in general was out of whack due to the prescription drugs I had been on for years, the processed foods I was eating, my emotional health, my lifestyle in general, and my entire past health history.

I met my husband, Life Lesson 4 (LL4), when I was 26 and he was 22. I was still a train wreck as far as my health and all my symptoms were concerned; I was getting worse even with new prescriptions. I entered my first fitness competition in 2001 since I had such a passion for dance performance and being on stage. I wasn't ready to give that up. The foods I was putting into my body changed again with this new venture, but I still had IBS. LL4 drank alcohol often and smoked while drinking. I had gone from age 21 to age 26 without smoking at all. I quit cold turkey. When I met him, I started smoking socially again if we were out drinking. Smoking still made me sick though, so it didn't last too long. I had reoccurring sinus infections which made me low on energy, and I coughed all the time. I still was on several prescription drugs which I thought was normal. I would get better temporarily, but symptoms would come back again. The drugs were masking my problems, not curing them. I would get the flu even though I had gotten the flu shot. The last time I had the flu was 2005 and that was the last time I had a flu shot as well. In 2006, I stumbled upon an integrative doctor, one who looks at the body as a whole and prescribes supplements and nutrition versus drugs. My health has never been better since I meet Dr. Turner and Dr. O' Brien of Turner Chiropractic Care. I had made an appointment to see them based on chronic PMS symptoms. Instead of giving me a cream or a supplement for my PMS they put me on a liver detox which was a medicinal shake. A few weeks into the regimen, I had a reaction; I started bleeding when I was going to the bathroom. Sorry if that is TMI (too much information), but with my personal training clients, nothing is TMI. The doctors then recommended a stool analysis, which I did. This sounds super gross, but truth be told, it can tell the amount and types of bacteria residing in your intestines and stomach. Yuck! Our guts house 75% of our immune system and most chronic disease and inflammation starts there. When I got the results back, we finally had a definitive answer to decades of my having been chronically sick: candida, gut dysbiosis; leaky gut! Plus, my flora was 85% bad bacteria and only 15% good bacteria, hence my always being so sick and not being able to fight off illness. Actually, our gut flora should be the reverse; 85% good bacteria and 15% bad.

Both doctors asked if I had been breast-fed, which I hadn't. They also had me look back at my health history since birth and recommended a book which really opened my eyes: *Gut and Psychology Syndrome* by Dr. Natasha Campbell-McBride, MD. I highly recommend reading it. Not having been breast-fed definitely had a negative impact on my immunity and led to a plethora of chronic conditions starting in my mid-teenage years. Plus, all the years of taking antibiotics created inflammation in my gut. Even the dates of my immunizations are linked to problems I was having from my senior year of high school into my early college years. It was at this time in my life that I questioned my mom on all of this and found out I was sick my first few weeks of life with an upper respiratory infection. My sterile baby gut was plugged full of antibiotics, so I didn't get a healthy start at life. Three months after my birth she noted I had a fever. Most people think all of this is normal, but it's not.

According to Campbell-McBride:

The most important thing that should happen is breastfeeding. Breast milk, particularly colostrum in the first days after birth, is vital for appropriate population of the baby's digestive system with healthy microbial flora. It is known that formula-fed babies develop completely different gut flora to breast-fed babies. That flora later on predisposes formula-fed babies to asthma, eczema, allergies and other health problems. Breast is best! However, if a woman/ mother has gut dysbiosis, the gut lining is leaky and damaged. Unhealthy parents produce unhealthy children.

Breast-feeding for two years might be considered a prolonged time by today's standards, but this practice offers significant protection against childhood diseases, including allergies and asthma. One recent study showed that breast-feeding for less than 9 months was found to be a risk factor for asthma and after that period of time, the longer the child was breast-fed, the lower the risk of asthma. Avoiding cow's milk proteins, even those found in infant formulas, has also been shown to reduce asthma occurrence.

Candida

What is Candida? It is the best known fungus to cause untold misery to millions. Candida Albicans is a yeast that lives inside of almost all of us. When it gets out of control, we call it a Candida overgrowth. This overgrowth of fungus in the body is much more common than you might think. Eeeww, right? A few things that cause Candida overgrowth include being on a series of antibiotics, eating sugar and starch often, drinking, smoking, and the list goes on. Candida feeds off sugar. I experienced 12 of these Candida symptoms for over two decades. Today, I rarely if ever experience any symptoms at all. If I do, it is because I decided to feed my body processed crap, drink alcohol, or experience some type of negative emotional stressor that I am not used to.

Symptoms of Candida

Fatigue*	**Sinus Congestion/ Infections***
Yeast Infections	**Bloating and Gas***
Joint Pain*	Weight Gain
Brain Fog	Urinary Infections
Frequent Colds*	**Food Cravings***
Oral Thrush	Irritability
Headaches	**Food Sensitivities***
Mood Swings*	Insomnia
Dizziness	**Abdominal Pain***
Itching	Red, Itchy Eyes
Acne*	Rashes Psoriasis/ Eczema Allergies

In bold are reoccurring symptoms I experienced over two decades. Most conventional doctors will prescribe medicine for any of these above symptoms, which will only mask them. To rid the body of these, individuals need to change what they are eating, what supplements they take, and even their lifestyle, which includes everything from sleep habits, to cooking food versus eating out.

"Did you know that Medical Error is the number three cause of death in the United States? Heart Disease and Cancer being number one and number two. 30% of healthcare spending (roughly $750 billion annually) is wasted and does not improve health." - Escape Fire: The Fight to Rescue American Healthcare, Susan Froemke and Matthew Heineman

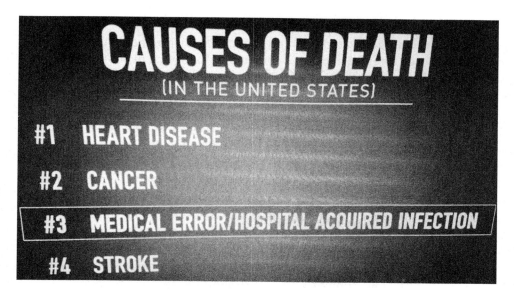

CAUSES OF DEATH
(IN THE UNITED STATES)

#1 HEART DISEASE

#2 CANCER

#3 MEDICAL ERROR/HOSPITAL ACQUIRED INFECTION

#4 STROKE

My integrative doctor prescribed a diet in which I had a list of approved foods and non-approved foods to choose from. I started introducing my body to new healthier foods. I was given about thirty supplements in total to take, three of which were crucial to my healing. My doctor prescribed a shelf stable high dose probiotic taken three times a day to increase my healthy "good" beneficial flora, an anti-Candida supplement that killed off the fungus, and an adrenal supplement to support and strengthen my adrenals. If you are always getting sick, most likely your adrenals are shot and your gut is a train wreck. Most conventional doctors don't look at these two very important organs, nor do they test for damage or weakness.

The first two months of following my plan 100%, I was tired every single day, and napping often which is part of the die-off/ detox symptoms; that means the fungus is being killed. My body was highly toxic. Most people don't realize that a person will feel worse before feeling better when doing a detox. Many people are not always able to push through a detox in hope of ridding their body of all the toxins that have accumulated over the years. Doing a detox is not easy. Die-off symptoms vary per individual. After seven months of sticking to my plan 100%, outside of having only one hamburger, bun included, one scoop of ice cream, and one Vodka soda in the middle of summer, I finally got relief! Yes, I stuck to it for seven months and consumed only those three items not on my plan. When you get to a point where you are sick of being sick, you'll do anything. If you can relate you are probably cheering reading this. After seven months, I retested and my stool analysis came back normal; no more Candida/gut dysbiosis and my flora was balanced, 85% good and 15% bad. I had seen the light at this point and there was no turning back. Ever since doing this detox, I no longer get ill like I used to, I no longer have Asthma, and the "I no longer" list goes on. Everyone's journey is different but I have referred several friends, family, and clients to my integrative doctor, and they too have gotten relief.

From this point on, I graduated to different types of testing and methods of healing. Just because I retested and saw a complete turn-around did not mean my journey to better health was over; it had only just begun! I later took an adrenal saliva test since I had been experiencing symptoms of adrenal dysfunction for most of my life. Dr. Turner also recommended Meridian Stress Assessment testing, which tests the strength of your organs and then recommends which supplements work best with your body to return the organ(s) to optimal function. In about a year, I was able to get great results with this as well. However, the three organs that seemed to be weak at that time were my adrenals, small intestine, and liver, which makes sense. Our liver is our filter, and my liver was stressed, especially with all the prescription drugs I had been on, along with the abuse I suffered for decades. My small intestine was negatively affected by all the drugs and not having been breast-fed. My adrenals were shot from so many stressors. I've had laser treatments for my adrenals periodically over the past ten years and these helped a lot when I felt bogged down. I still take supplements that support my adrenals to this day. We all experience stress throughout our lives, so getting over one hump doesn't mean you'll never be stressed again. I learned that my body and I are a team; I am my own scientist. I am more aware of how my body feels, and more aware of my emotions which have a huge impact on our health. I can now tell when things are off in my body so I don't wait until it's too late, backpedaling, like most Americans do. I practice preventative medicine and get in to see my trusted integrative doctor as soon as possible to get relief at the first sign of symptoms. I still see Dr. Turner yearly for maintenance check-ups and supplements, especially when I am bogged down with stress.

What are your adrenals and why are they important?

"The adrenal glands are two small glands, each about the size of an acorn, that sit at the top of both kidneys. They are responsible for secreting important hormones, including cortisol, that help the body respond to stress. Many of us are living lives full of stressful events — work, family, commuting, relationships, finances and more. All this stress may cause our adrenal glands to work overtime, leading to what is often called adrenal fatigue, or adrenal exhaustion. This can lead to a lack of energy, weight gain, sugar cravings, and reliance on stimulants like caffeine to get moving every day."
-TerryTalksNutrition.com

Adrenal dysfunction is more widespread than people think and most conventional doctors don't know how to test or treat it. The majority of my clients show symptoms of adrenal dysfunction. I then prescribe adrenal saliva testing for them as well (we offer it at the gym I work for) to better determine supplementation and other lifestyle changes necessary to repair them. Getting to the root cause and implementing long-term dietary changes and supplements will cure it. Attached is a chart of causes of adrenal dysfunction symptoms from *Adrenal Fatigue, The 21st Century Stress Syndrome* by James L. Wilson.

FACTORS AFFECTING THE ADRENALS

Financial Pressure · Death of a Loved One · Repeated Stresses · Psychological Stress · Toxins · Infection Acute & Chronic · Emotional Stress · Lack Of Relaxation · Allergies · Negative Attitudes & Beliefs · Over Excertion · Unwanted Unemployment · Smoking · Fear · Lack of Sleep · Coffee · Poor Eating Habits · Caffeine · Sugar & White Flour Products · Lack of Good Food · Lack of, or Excessive Excercise · Marital Stress · Perscription, Non-perscription Drugs · Wound Healing

Allergies	Respiratory disorders
Fatigue	Re-occurring infections
Arthritis	Insomnia
Depression	Constipation
Diarrhea	Weight gain
Cravings for salt or sugar	Cravings for carbohydrates and fat
Reliance on sugar and caffeine	Intolerance to cold
Low blood pressure	Low stamina for stress
Lightheadedness upon standing up	Fainting or Faintness
Hair loss	Acne
Mental Depression	Moodiness
Nervousness	Neck or Trapezius muscle pain
Lack of libido	Excessive sweating from little activity
Weakness	Heart palpitations
Waking up feeling fatigued even after sufficient number of hours of sleep	Sleep disturbances (feeling wired at night, waking up frequently)

Now, back to more on Candida. Research has shown that 70% of us have Candida in our guts, so why isn't everyone talking about Candida overgrowth? It's a difficult condition for conventional doctors to diagnose because the symptoms are so difficult to pin down. Many people go through much of their adult lives without getting a proper diagnosis from their doctors. Headaches and fatigue become "just a part of normal life," joint pain is written off as a symptom of "getting old," and depression or mood swings are simply endured. This doesn't have to be the case, though. You can get relief and rid your body of this condition with healing foods from the land and sea along with the right supplementation dosage and other lifestyle changes.

Interview with Dr. Turner

When I first met Nicole, it was a bit of work to find the base of her chronic health problems. This was not the first time I had seen this, but it does take time to get to the root. I helped write a book called <u>Performance Without Pain</u> with a patient of mine who was a professional musician. This was when I made the connection between gastrointestinal tracts and the stomach inflammation that can be manifested.

This is a pain that comes and goes, and it can range from a 10 to a 3 while a person lives in some form of discomfort all the time. People with this type of pain are more than qualified to be disabled due to the level of pain; however, the government does not see this yet as something that would put a person on that sort of list.

On the surface, Nicole never let this slow her down. She never let it shape her, but the pain she endured would have disabled most people. I think that due to her ability to focus, she was able to deal with it better than most. My professional viewpoint about how she has dealt with this is that she is amazing; most people would not be able to manage their lives the way Nicole does. Nicole lives a more than normal life; she is a high achiever.

One thing I would like people to know about Nicole is that on the surface she is talented and beautiful, and she looks like she has had an easy life but it's really just the opposite: she does not take things for granted. She's had to work harder than most to get where she is. What Nicole deals with is manageable but not curable. Had she not put forth the time and hard work, she would not be a healthy person free of years of chronic symptoms.

Serving as a personal trainer and a holistic health advocate is not an easy life to begin with. You're a coach, a trainer, and an example as to what peoples' goals might be. This is very difficult to do on a daily basis. She sets the standards high for all her clients based on all she has achieved herself.

We spent some time together when her mom passed. As far as being head strong goes, on a scale of 1-10, she is a 12. She is amazingly able to deal with pain, both mentally and physically. I would have understood if she had thrown in the towel. Most people would have. She has taken control of her life, and more importantly, her health, and for that I applaud her.

To know what she had to overcome to get to where she is at in the business is amazing within itself. The type of discipline she has is a moment to mo-

ment thing as in "will this get me closer to health or will this take my future away?" She maximizes every moment of every day.

I personally felt great to know her, and see Nicole walk the stage at the Bikini Olympia 2012. We spent a lot of time together getting her health back on track. The emotional, physical, and chemical stress from the foods she was eating and all the prescriptions drugs she had taken created a long road to poor health. We worked really hard together to reverse that. While I feel like I am part of the team, she still did the work.

Leaky Gut

"A body fed correctly, not poisoned via diet, modern medicine, fast and processed food, does not break down. Anyone arguing is brainwashed." - Roger Bezanis

The pharmaceutical industry, aka "Big Pharma", does NOT create cures; it creates customers. I have LGS (leaky gut syndrome) as do many, and it goes misdiagnosed in western medicine. For your reference, I wanted to include "Symptoms, Causes and Solutions" by Heather Gardner:

Could Leaky Gut be the source of all those nagging health concerns?

Did you ever wonder why you have so many strange health conditions that just don't go away? And no matter how many times you go for a check-up, get a massage, do hot yoga, and gulp down green smoothies, that bloated tummy, drippy nose, bad skin, and brain fog just won't budge? Isn't it just annoying when your friends and family are chugging coffee, downing doughnuts, and digging into deep fried everything and for some reason you seem to feel worse than they do?

Well instead of throwing in the towel after yet another Pilates® class, know that there are solutions out there when you know what is causing the problem. Leaky gut and candida, often related, can cause all sorts of different health problems, and as a result can go undetected for years. But if you educate yourself about these problems and their solutions, you can be sitting pretty once more and striding with a spring in your step!

Undigested protein molecules in the small intestine can create holes and cause inflammation. Once that happens, the undigested protein can get into the bloodstream. If you have protein in the bloodstream, the body recognizes it as a foreign invader and starts to attack it. This can cause auto immune diseases, such as hives, eczema, mental fog, or fatigue, joint pain, swelling, or arthritis. Food allergies are a key sign.

Some Common Symptoms of Leaky Gut

Hives, eczema, mental fog, or fatigue, joint pain, swelling, or arthritis. Food allergies, sinus or nasal congestion, especially shortly after you eat. Chronic or frequent inflammation anywhere in your body, injuries or sores that don't heal quickly. Confusion, poor memory, or mood swings. Bowel diseases like colitis, Crohn's disease, and celiac disease.

Conditions Associated with Leaky Gut Syndrome

Accelerated Aging	Celiac disease	Endotoxemia	Malnutrition
Acne	Chemotherapy	Fibromyalgia	Multiple Chemical Sensitivities
AIDS	Chronic Fatigue Syndrome	Food allergies	Multiple Sclerosis
Alcoholism	Chronic hepatitis	Food Intolerance	Pancreatic dysfunction
Ankylosing Spondylitis	Colon cancer	Giardia	Psoriasis
Arthritis	Crohn's disease	Hives	Schizophrenia
Asthma	Cystic Fibrosis	Inflammatory bowel disease	Ulcerative Colitis
Autism	Dermatitis	Irritable Bowel Syndrome	
Candidiasis	Eczema	Liver dysfunction	

Not eating in a relaxed frame of mind, eating on the run, while at work, or when stressed. Not chewing properly. Having low stomach acid. Not having enough enzymes in the diet or repeatedly eating enzyme depleting cooked foods. Bad food combining. Eating damaging foods such as processed foods. Partially digested food particles. Overworked and stressed pancreas, liver, and gallbladder. Eating processed grains, sugar, and alcohol. Smoking. The measles vaccine.

Leaky Gut Prevention and Cure Action Steps

- Digestion begins in the mind; relax before eating.
- Chew until your food is liquid.
- Practice food combining; avoid protein and sweet combinations, fruit and oil combinations.
- Eat plenty of raw food to increase enzymes.
- Drink at least 2 liters of water a day away from meal times. You can have it warm, with some lemon, or with pinches of green superfood powders.
- Remove processed foods and recreational drugs, cigarettes, and coffee.
- Leave long gaps between meals--at least 4 hours--and replace some meals with green juice.
- Plan some 'liquid only' days to give the body a break.

Supplements to Help Heal Leaky Gut

- Flax (ground)/ chia (whole) gel
- Chia Seeds
- Slippery Elm
- Licorice
- Acidophilus/ probiotics
- Digestive Enzymes
- Glutamine
- Ginger
- Zinc
- Quercetin
- Turmeric
- Marshmallow root
- Aloe Vera
- Plantain
- Propolis
- Calendula

Foods to Help Heal Leaky Gut

- Animal fat, lard, tallow
- Dandelion greens and green leafy vegetables
- Jicama, artichoke, chicory and dandelion
- Fermented foods
- Sauerkraut, kefir, kimchi
- Coconut oil and other tropical oils
- Chamomile

How to Heal the Gut

Remove inflammatory foods from the diet.

Use digestive enzymes to enhance assimilation of food and to create an ideal pH within the gut.

De-inflame the digestive lining and lay down nutrients to tighten up the gap junctions (holes) of the digestive tract. Healthy fats and fermented foods are best for this.

Build up the villi which increases the surface area of the intestines.

Lay down antibodies and probiotics to strengthen our first line immune defense.

I personally would like to add in and really stress the importance of consuming healthy fats daily as a prescription to repairing a leaky gut. I work with clients today on getting a variety of healthy fats into their menus.

Over the years, I have had major food bullies in my life; most of my clients and fit friends do too. It's a conversation I typically have with all of them at one point or another. We just want to be left alone with our food. I don't question someone else's weight or what's on their plate. Why pick on me? Leave me and my healthy food choices alone. Okay, rant over. Most people make poor choices with food. When the heart attack comes, they always wonder why. I've learned that it is difficult to be healthy in an unhealthy world.

I started my journey in 2006 and it's never-ending. I am continually tweaking, eliminating, and adding new things to my meal plan. I have my tribe of experts I reach out to; Dr. Turner, Dr. Schuster of Total Athleticare, Karyn Calabrese of Karyn's Raw (in Chicago), Alyce Sorokie of Partners in Wellness (also in Chicago), Corey Kelly, Donna Ichikawa and John Newton to name a few. I notice much relief with every change I make. Just know that if you too suffer from the same, there is no instant fix. It's a twenty mile hike every day, but for me, my quality of life now versus then has been worth it all. People see me and say, "Oh you look so good!

You're healthy." The main point of this chapter and sharing my health history is that the gym did not turn my health around for the better. Changing what I put into my body daily did. Eating better, cooking food instead of eating out, getting off all prescription drugs, thinking better, working on myself instead of blaming others, eliminating toxic people, and the list goes on; doing all this is when my health turned around for the better.

"He who cures a disease may be the skillfullest, but he that prevents it, is the safest physician." - Thomas Fuller

Chapter 4 - Life Lessons

"The more difficulty that Allah is putting on you right now, the more tests you're getting, and the greater you will become, so embrace those tests. Yes, you might have some difficulties. No, things are not easy, and yes, there are obstacles in life, but realize that those difficulties prepare you to be an amazing person. The more difficult things become in your life, the greater you will become, so try not to complain. Try not to feel that Allah doesn't love you. He is only preparing you. This is just like when you're in a weight room. If you lift only one bar, if you only run for three minutes, you're not going to lose a lot of weight. How are you going to get strong? How are you going to get in shape? Only if you do a lot of work. Allah is telling you to work now because you're going to become great. Each and every one of you has the potential of becoming great. It's just the way you see your problems." - Saqema A., my best friend since diapers, who is Muslim; we are going on 42 years of friendship.

Life Lesson #1 aka LL1

It's amazing how the first heartbreak changes your outlook on every relationship after that.

In high school, I dated guys here and there for a few weeks at a time, but nothing serious. During junior year, the guy who sat behind me in math class was always flirting with me. We ended up becoming very good friends. He later became Life Lesson #1 (LL1). He sucked at math and he cheated off me on tests. While I was getting an A in class sophomore year, I ended up getting an F on the final because I let LL1 cheat off me on the final test. We got caught, so I ended up with a B. He had a C going into the final and ended up with a D. He asked me out often, and I always said no. When the King of Hearts dance came around junior year (it's when the girl asks the guy to the dance), I asked him to go. He, of course, said yes. We then started dating after the dance for two and a half years. We also went to college together briefly but we did break up freshman year. At the beginning things were great; however, our relationship ended up quite tumultuous. During the 2 1/2 years we dated, I caught LL1 cheating on me 8 times, and yet, dummy me, I still stayed with him and kept going back. I was young--16 years old; I did not know better seeing it was my first long-term relationship. I gave a lot to him and our relationship.

A month or two into dating, we were at a party, and we had a disagreement. I got mad and left. He ended up kissing his ex-girlfriend. I found out the next day when he told me, "Oh, I was drunk. I thought it was you." She is blonde and looked nothing like me. This was just one of many examples. I was the captain and MVP of the Pom Squad senior year, and he was the captain of the basketball team. He also played baseball. He was used to being in the spotlight. I was too. His eldest brother played for the NBA at the time we dated. LL1 never did make it to a professional sports team. He was very controlling and possessive when we dated. He did not like me wearing make-up or styling my hair. I pretty much had to wear a garbage bag to make him happy. I could not wear anything that showed off my body. Each time we broke up, it would only be for one night, and then he would make out with another girl for that night, saying it was OK since we had broken up for that day or night. He cheated on me with a girl who was my best friend at the time. We'll call her Douche Bag # 1, aka DBAG1. I'll get to that story later; it happened after our senior prom. There was one time when DBAG1 and I went shopping at the mall. Afterwards, I met LL1 at a friend's house; it was not a party, but a get-together. I arrived late, and when I arrived, I was told that LL1 was upstairs getting high and that he wanted me to go to McDonald's to get him some fries. So I was like, OK, and I left, thinking nothing of it. DBAG1 and I left to get his fries and when we returned, he came down and ate his fries. I got to school that week and an-other girl that was there that night told me that LL1 was upstairs "with" another girl: DBAG2 (a best friend from my younger years; we took dance class together and played all the time during our grade school years). When I went to get the fries, he kicked DBAG2 out. To this day, I am guarded around many women and even men. I am grateful for all the honest people in my life today. However, I have had to weed a lot of people out over the decades. Right after this girl told me about DBAG2, LL1 walked up and met me at my locker like usual. He was next to me, and DBAG2 was across the hall at her locker. I called him out on it in front of everyone. I told him, "You lied to me. You were with her when you made me go and get fries." Well, my standing my ground and not putting up with his crap did-n't last long. He snaked his way back into my life. Mind you again, I was only 16, and it was my first long-term relationship.

At NCA Pom Camp during the summer of 1989, I won the opportunity to perform in the 1989 Macy's Day Thanksgiving Day Parade. I remember two things about this once-in-a-lifetime event: getting on the school bus heading home and saying goodbye to LL1 before heading to NYC. He was so mean to me! I always supported him on everything, and I was so upset with how mean he was to me. Then my dad never said goodbye or wished me well before I left for NYC. He did not even watch me on television! It's happened many times in my life that men, including my own father, could not be happy for me, my successes, and my accomplishments. It hurts. When you are dating someone or married and he/she is not there for you, it's a horrible feeling; being alone with no support even though you are with some-one especially when you are experiencing exciting things yourself. I do remember that my mom was there for me. She took me to the airport and told me to have fun and not worry about either of them. She always supported me no matter what I did. She watched me on television on Thanksgiving morning. She tape recorded it, and bragged to everyone that she saw me on NBC. We all need more cheerleaders in our lives. At 42, I am still a cheerleader for life, with my clients, my friends, and my family. My mom was my cheerleader, so I had the best example.

I went to senior prom with LL1. He and I were hanging out together at the dance, and DBAG1 had gone with someone else. For some odd reason (which didn't really click until much later), she was hanging around us most of the night. I was getting a weird vibe; my gut instinct told me something was going on between them by their interactions with one another. A week or so later I had heard rumors and people were telling me things about the two of them being together behind my back. I spoke with her, and she lied. She said no, and that she loved me and would never do that. I asked him, and at that time he lied to me too and said no. DBAG1 has never admitted to me that she was with LL1 behind my back, not even to this day. She even got her mom involved and had her call my mom. I ended up having to go to DBAG1's house to apologize to her for not believing her; my mom made me do this. It all came out around a year later that they were together, sexually. LL1 came clean and admitted this to me as well as her best friend in her grade; DBAG1 was a year younger than we were. DBAG1 is an only child. We often spent the holidays at her house playing games, taking vacations together, and doing all sorts of fun things. I do miss her parents; they are amazing. I even got her on the Pom Squad without her having to audition. She had a math contest that same day as tryouts and was unable to attend. Yes, I had that kind of pull, even in high school. My coaches loved and trusted me, which was a big mistake. She was a horrible dancer and the girls on the squad were pissed off at me for asking the coaches to allow her on the squad without auditioning like the rest of the girls. They all said she should not be on the squad; that is how bad she was.

"What is bullying? – It's not just physical.

Lying to get you in trouble
Threats and name-calling
Spreading rumors (story of my life)
Stealing your belongings"

   - Don't Wait Project, Lisa Bradshaw

I share some stories later of being bullied as an adult by DBAG3 and DBAG5.

We really don't lose friends. We just kind of discover who our real friends are. LLI and I went to Iowa State University together. Before we started, he had already expressed to me that he did not like a few things about college. It was hard for him leaving high school where he was well known by all to attend college where he was a newbie. He did not like the baseball team either, the reason he attended Iowa State. He arrived at school a few weeks early to start training with the team. He was miserable before I got there when school started. The first week of college freshman year, I went out to a frat party with my female best friend from high school. I ended up meeting this super cute guy, and he asked me out on a date. I accepted his invitation, so we went out for pizza during week two. Things between

LL1 and me were not going well at the time. Wait, were they ever? The guy kissed me after dinner. It was not a make out kiss or anything; it was just a peck. I felt horrible. I had not been with anybody in the 2.5 years LL1 and I had dated, yet he had been with several girls behind my back. A day or so later, LL1 and I started arguing and somehow it came out that I went on this date. Now, keep in mind he already was unhappy at college, but because I kissed another guy, he left school and dropped out, blaming it on me and how hurt he was. Look at the pot calling the kettle black! He got a dose of his own medicine, which didn't taste good. I told him I kissed a guy, and he left college; went home. I was the excuse for him not staying there. It's always easier to blame another. Personally, I don't think he was ready for college at that time based on all he had shared with me regarding how unhappy he was prior to my kiss.

Believe it or not, we still dated after that, and at that point I did find out that he was with DBAG1. Fast forward to summer, the first summer after freshman year of college. He had a party (he held parties often). We were arguing in his back yard; it could have been about the fact I was wearing a mini-skirt. It was a total high school/ teenage relationship. I was smoking a cigarette while we were arguing. At the time I smoked if I was drinking or studying. He was yelling and saying some very mean things to me. He slapped the cigarette out of my hand, called me a name, and I slapped him. He punched me in my face which bruised my cheek. I ended up running inside his house and getting my best friend, and we left immediately. We went down the street to another party where I had parked my car. When I left this party to head home, my tires were all flat. Someone had removed the air in my tires. How ironic! I knew it was LL1. I called the police and they helped put air in my tires. The police saw the bruise, and I ended up taking him to court for battery. As a result, he had to do some community service. We did not talk for a year after that. He ended up going to a community college, then off to a four year college, and later moved to another state.

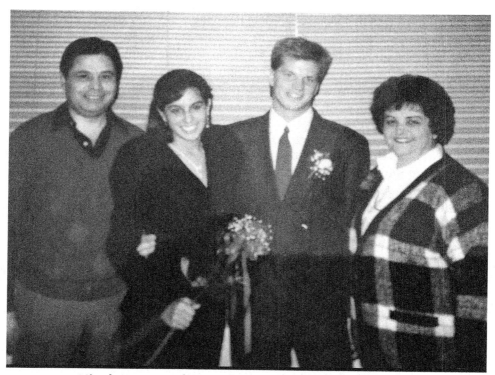

Nicole Moneer (Center Left) and LL#1 (Center Right)

In 2004, he contacted me via email on my website. He wrote a long apology email admitting his faults and wrongdoings while we dated in high school back in 1989-1991, almost 13 years earlier. Better late than never, eh? At the time I received his email, I was engaged to be married. LL1 told me he had been going through the yearbook, had reread what I wrote to him our senior year, and felt horrible for how he had mistreated me. He told me that if I ever wanted to talk, he was there for me. I did call him, and we made amends; it was good. I needed that--his apology. He took ownership for how he had mistreated me and taken me for granted. We made peace between us via a telephone conversation. I am always open to accept someone's apology and talk things out. If you hold on to anger (which I did for many years) it messes you up, not just mentally, but physically. Toxic emotions that we harbor can negatively impact our health. My relationship with LL1 messed me up for a long time, even in my marriage. If you have the power to apologize and forgive, life gets so much easier. It took me awhile to master both, although I still work on both to this day.

In relationships #3 and #4, I was very insecure and continued asking the "why?" questions: "Why are you talking to that girl?" "Why do you pay more attention to her than you do to me?" I carried this--not trusting people--with me for over a decade, since I had been betrayed by LL1 so many times, and later LL2. LL1 came into town during the summer of 2005 and contacted me. We went out with another girlfriend of mine and had a blast. Nothing happened, sexually that is. We hung out as friends and had a good time. Today, he and I are still friends. We were young, and yes, he was a punk at the time but his apology did help me heal tremendously in my marriage. Plus, it felt good to forgive him. Often we carry things with us thinking there is something wrong with us, that we aren't good enough or something of that sort, **when really it is the person who cheats who is not fulfilled and trying to fill a void.**

There were issues that came up later in my marriage that were tied to this. It is sad that in life sometimes people never get the apology they need to move on. Often, we need to learn to forgive those who hurt us anyway, which is difficult to do. I always thought there was something wrong with me. I was cheated on and mistreated, which had nothing to do with me and everything to do with him. I learned this much later in marital counseling in 2005. When people react or dump their problems on you, it has to do with them or their past, often their childhood and how they were treated, but it takes two to tango. There is no sense in escalating a situation by getting your shit mixed in with the other person's. Then the only thing you end up with is a big pile of shit. Excuse my French, but it's the truth and a great way to get my point across. People who have been hurt, hurt other people. Today LL1 is a business owner and we are friends. My publisher interviewed LL1. Read on (below) to see what he had to say. I was very touched.

Life Lesson #1 Phone Interview

Nicole and I are close friends today. We took a long time off from one another. This being said, I love her to death, and she is one of the sweetest people I have met. We dated in high school and briefly in college too. We went through some tough times. We were kids. While we were young kids, we still loved one another. We dated for 2.5 years, 20 years ago. We took about 11 years without talking, then I contacted her via email. Then one night we talked on the phone, and it was like we never missed a beat. It was easy to become friends again due to her positive outlook on life. It was very refreshing, and hard to accept. She is a very positive person, and one of the most positive people I have ever met too.

One thing I would like people to know is how strong minded she is and how genuine a person she is as well. You see a lot of people in her business, and there is a lot of talk and they don't do what they say they are going to do. She does not say something to get 10,000 likes on Facebook; she means what she says.

We went to every dance together junior and senior year. There was not much we did not do. We did everything together and in my high school

41

year book she wrote on the whole back page. To this day it is still the nicest, sweetest thing anyone has said about me. Back in high school, I played sports and my brother played sports too. The one thing I never lacked was confidence, and she wrote that. I still have never heard people talk like that. It's not something she just started doing; she always was a coach.

She means what she says, like Tony Robbins with his Colgate smile who gets paid to make you feel good about yourself.

Life Lesson #2 aka LL2

"Every failed relationship is an opportunity for self-growth and learning. Be thankful and move on!" - @ihatequotes via Twitter

My mom always stuck up for any guy I brought home, which leads me to LL2. My dad never approved of anyone. Aren't most fathers like this with their daughters? My dad did not approve of me dating LL2 period. LL2's doctor knew my dad. His doctor told my dad, "Your daughter is way too good for him," along with other patient/doctor confidential information he should have never shared with my father. We met at a party my sophomore year in college during the summer. We had good times together, but just the typical relationship of someone in their late teens, early twenties.

Before I go on, I need to interject with DBAG3. During my internship at Nordstrom during the summer of 1993, I met a girl who was a World Champion Chicago Bulls Cheerleader. We had a great conversation upon meeting. I told her I was attending the Luvabull camp prior to the auditions. At camp we learned a few dances and received some pointers from the coach, Cathy Core. She let each of us know if there was anything we needed to work on or change before auditioning. For example, she told me I needed more mascara and to wax my brows; easy stuff for me to change. Other girls were told they needed to lose weight, remove their braces, and the like. I remember coming into work after attending the camp and DBAG3 comes up to me asking about some blonde who looked like Marilyn Monroe that attended camp and saying how the coach really liked her. I felt pretty confident walking away from that camp. I had nailed the dance routines, and Cathy had advised some easy changes for me to make for the audition. After DBAG3 said all this to me about that blonde, I felt like she was trying to intimidate me and make me feel as if I was not good enough for the squad. Anyway, I did later make the 1994-1995 World Champion Chicago Bulls Cheerleaders, The Luvabulls. DBAG3 even went as far as to inform my boss at Nordstrom that I made the squad before I could tell her. Pretty shady! I had already discussed "making the squad" with my boss and asked her that if I did make the team, would it be a problem to have two nights off for rehearsals and also for game days. My boss had said that DBAG3 was rarely at work, and that if and when I made the squad, we would further discuss it;

we--not DBAG3 and her. I come to find out, DBAG3 had bad mouthed me to the staff at Nordstrom and to the veterans on The Luvabulls. It then made sense as to why so many of these girls were cold and mean to me when I would approach them, talk to them, or even compliment them. DBAG3 was making up lies about me behind my back. Why? I had never done anything to her; I barely knew her. It was jealousy, I am guessing. However, DBAG3 also lied to our boss; she would erase her name off the Nordstrom Brass Plum schedule without getting approval, just so she could cheer at games and work other paid appearances, hence, my boss saying that she was never there. Ironically, after I made the 1994-1995 Luvabulls, DBAG3 quit Nordstrom. Another Luvabull and a Nordstrom employee filled me in on all the lies DBAG3 had said behind my back a few weeks after she quit, and a few weeks after I made the squad.

Going back to LL2, in 1994, LL2 was over at my house. My dad came home from work, saw us, and right in front of LL2 he said, "I told you he is not welcome in our home." After that, my dad did not talk with me for two years. He never even sat down and had a conversation with me during this time to explain why he did not want LL2 in the house or dating me. My father also did not speak with my mom during this time either. However, that was typical of their thirty year marriage. They divorced in January of 1996. My mom later told me that my dad had spoken with LL2's doctor, and that LL2's doctor told my dad that he was not the right person for his (my dad's) daughter based on his chemical dependencies/addictions and some other trouble with the law he had gotten into prior to our time together dating.

I was about 20 when LL2 and I started dating, and we were together until I was about 22. He had a drinking problem, but at the time it didn't affect us, well, at least not until the end of our relationship. I was not dating him to marry him; we simply had fun together. My mom loved every guy that was in my life, and every boyfriend of mine loved my mom. She would cook them dinner or take them out to dinner. She accepted everyone, girlfriends included. She accepted me 110%. My mom stood up for LL2. He did a lot for my mom; he helped her with her business and did other odds and ends around the house. I was hired as a Chicago Bulls Cheerleader for the 1994-1995 season, and during this time I was dating LL2. For each game I cheered, I would get two complimentary tickets which I would give to friends and family. When I worked a game, I would have to be there two hours before the game began. LL2 was attending a game with a guy friend of mine from work, so he needed to pick him up and drive him to the game. LL2 had met him since I got him a job at my work; off topic, he messed that up as well. This is one of the reasons why I am hesitant to put in a good word for people. Each time I refer or recommend someone for a job, they screw up, which makes me look bad in the end, but back to the game day story. So LL2 never showed up at my work (Nordstrom) to pick up my guy friend nor did he even go to work that day, so my two Bulls tickets went to waste. I did not find out the truth behind this story until after LL2 and I broke up.

Before we broke up, my godmother came into town and my mom bought tickets on the floor behind the players' bench for them to attend the game at which I was cheering. LL2 was attending this game with one of my best friend's mom, using my two tickets which were in a different section. When they got to "will call" to pick up their two tickets, will call messed up and told them the tickets I had for them were not there. Since they had driven downtown to the United Center already, they just bought tickets, but ended up sitting separately since they were only able to find single tickets. LL2 was in a different section of the United Center that night making new friends. He got very drunk at this game. When the game was over, I don't remember exactly what he did but he was very disrespectful to my mom in front of all of us. She did nothing but stick up for him in front of my father and did so many nice things for him during the time we dated. He and I left the game. I was going to take LL2 home. However, I took a bit of a detour after how rude he was to my mom! I know this city very well so instead of taking him home, I dropped him off at the hotel where we Luvabulls practiced. I took him some place safe, in case he reacted harshly. I kicked him out of the car there and left him in the city. I told him I never wanted to see him again for the way he had mistreated my mom. Sound cuckoo on my part? Just wait, it gets better! This was his karma, and I didn't know it at the time!

A week later, he was doing all he could to get back into my life. Around this same time, my coach from Luvabulls told me we needed to talk. She had received a let-ter from the head of the Bulls, her boss, and she read it to me. The head of the Bulls received a letter from a fan. This fan was handicapped and this fan and their significant other sat with LL2 in the handicap section during that game. So through-out the game, LL2 made friends with the couple, promised them tickets to another Bulls game and even gave them my cell number. Remember, he was drunk! So my coach wanted a letter of apology from him to her boss and this Bulls fan. When you're part of a team and people are sitting in seats, Luvabulls seats, they are a reflection of you. This is something our coach had said over and over again to us. Make sure whoever uses your tickets are responsible and respectful while in the stands, and that they do not tarnish your image. LL2 was begging to get back into my life, so I was like OK, and played along with it. I told him to take care of the let-ter to the Bulls and that we would move forward after that. He wrote the apology letter and did whatever he needed to do to make things right between us. As soon as I received his letters, I told him I was done. I had no intention of making amends with him. A few weeks later, I ended up meeting LL3. LL2 was still trying to get back with me, but after some time he finally left me alone. Now back to why he blew off that one game, which I found out after we broke up. He did not pick up my work friend and go to the Bulls game that night because he was with another girl, sexu-ally. Thus, in my first two long-term relationships, I was cheated on.

Life Lesson #3 aka LL3

"Being in a relationship is a full time job, so don't apply if you're not ready."
- Unknown

This brings us to LL3. He went to Iowa State where I went to college. When I was dating LL2, one of my sorority sisters had told me LL3 had a crush on me. At that time, I had no interest since I was with someone else. I later returned to college to celebrate Veishea in 1995, which was a weeklong celebration that happened every spring on campus. This time, I saw LL3 at a party, but I was single, so we ended up talking and hitting it off. Long story short, he moved to Chicago to date me and further his career. My father had moved out of our home at this point since my parents were going through a divorce, so my mom said LL3 could live with us and pay rent until he could find a place of his own, which he did.

I did audition to cheer for the Bulls again. I nailed all of the routines. The "vets" did auditions in camp and we did not have to go through the first few cuts like all the rookies. When I auditioned the previous year, I made the first day of cuts out of 250 some girls and then the final cut as well. I always made weigh-ins, and I had never been cut from working a game during the 1994-1995 season. Girls would get cut from a game if they did not make weight, broke out with pimples, forgot a uniform/ wardrobe while at a game, etc. There were five squads so we did not work every game like the players did. Each squad would have to audition for every game. Our coach was tough. If you didn't perform the routine well, she would remove you and add someone else who did. Out of the 14 rookies, there were only 4 of us that never got cut that year; I was one of them. So when I got cut from the 1995-1996 season auditions, I was in shock. I, along with another girl, did not make it back that year and we were crying our eyes out. We felt like the biggest losers, crying in the halls at the hotel where we rehearsed and auditioned.

At the time, I had been dating LL3 for about two months. He had lost his father a year before meeting me. We had gotten pretty serious, and he would have wanted me to meet his father but knew that would never happen since he was deceased. He missed his dad quite a bit. I remember talking with his mom when I did not make the Luvabulls again. His mom was so sweet; I really loved her. I remember her specifically saying to me that this was a good thing and that now LL3 could focus on me and supporting me which would take his mind off his father's death. Isn't this true? Helping others really helps us individually, and in the end, we often feel better. She often made us sweet treats (her caramel brownies were my favorite; they also did not help my gut health). At that time in my life I ate anything I wanted. I would just work it off in the gym. However, I was always super sick. I never was able to pin-point foods as being the main culprit of my chronic health problems until later when I hit my thirties.

I did get the opportunity to cheer for Michael Jordan while with the Luvabulls. He came out of retirement in March of 1995 and that was my game to work. When I cheered, back in the day, there was not an empty seat in the house. You could feel the energy and excitement. What a thrill! I would get goose-bumps every time we performed during the starting line-up. During the time LL3 and I dated, we ended up living together, not just at my mom's house, but once he moved out on his own, I moved in with him. I was in my early to mid-twenties in the four years we dated. At that time, I was all about myself, going out on the town with my girlfriends every weekend. Aren't our twenties the selfish years? I worked out, but at that time I did more cardio than weights. I was a cardio queen. I lived for aerobics classes; hi/ lo, step, double step, running, and hip hop funk classes. Does that show my age? LL3 and I worked out together at the same gym. We did a lot together; however, I often pushed him away to go out with "just the girls." He treated me like a queen and wanted to be with me as much as possible. I, on the other hand, liked my freedom. I wonder, was it the Sagittarius in me or my age and the fact that I did not appreciate what I had right in front of me at the time? Or maybe I had my guard up from past relationships?

I took LL3 to a family wedding in June of 1996. My dad was there since it was his best friend's daughter (my BBF of 42 year's older sister) who was getting married. My dad had not spoken to me for over two years because he thought I was still dating LL2. Remember him? My father met LL3 at the wedding and then he actually came up and spoke to me. He asked if he could take me shopping that week to buy a new car. I did not receive an apology for him not speaking with me for years and no explanation; just "let me buy you." This is how it was pretty much my whole life. It could be one reason why it took me until my thirties to learn how to say the words, "I am sorry." I never had a good example. Nor did I ever see my parents apologize to one another after a fight or a period of time where they did not speak to one another. This could also be why I have a hard time accepting gifts from others, especially men. I think they may take away whatever they bought me or hold it against me like my dad would do.

On Sunday June 9th, 1996 my dad's best friend had called my mom. I remember everything about this day. My mom and I had already moved out of my childhood home where I had lived for 23 years. LL3 had moved out and was living about thirty minutes away from us. We hadn't moved in together yet. I was in the middle of packing my gym bag for after work on Monday. My dad's friend had told my mom that we needed to get to the hospital because our father was there and it was an emergency. When we arrived he told us that my dad was dead. I still remember seeing my dad dead on the table. I can envision it now. I also remember the army of close friends and family who came to the ER that night. LL3 was my rock. He had been through it already with the death of his father. He was my "everything" during a very difficult time. I did not sleep a wink that night. I did not sleep much the first week, nor did I eat much the first week, and I did not work out.

My parents' divorce finalized in January, six months prior to his death. My dad's will was not updated. The last time it had been updated was almost ten years prior. Ironically, he was planning to update it the week after his unexpected death. Needless to say, my brother and I were next of kin and made executors of his estate. However, since my brother lived in San Diego, I was responsible for most of his estate. My dad was Muslim but did not practice his faith until later in life. My parents were married in a Catholic church, and my brother and I were raised Catholic. On Monday, we went to the funeral home to make arrangements. It was just awful for me. Muslims and Jews wake the deceased quickly. My mother and LL3 accompanied me to the funeral home. When we were discussing our preferences for his wake and funeral, a Muslim Imam was in the room. He had known my dad but none of us had ever met the Imam. He was arguing with us on what needed to be done based on Muslim tradition. My dad had just died the night before, and here was this Muslim stranger arguing with us? My father's will stated that he wanted to be embalmed and have an open casket. The Muslim priest chimed in and stated that in the Muslim community they don't embalm dead bodies and it's always a closed casket. They wrap the body in a shroud in a closed casket and wake the body immediately. My brother was in San Diego, CA trying to get a flight home to see his deceased father. He needed closure, so there was no way we were having a closed casket. I was fighting with the Imam that I didn't even know about all this crap. I did not need to be dealing with this. It was ridiculous and horrible to be fighting about the final wishes that we, as a family, had regarding the last time we would see our father. Furthermore, we remembered our dad in a suit; he always wore a suit to work.

In the end, we compromised. My father was embalmed, then wrapped in a shroud with an open casket. His closest Muslim friends bathed him, that is what they do in the Muslim faith, then they embalmed him and wrapped him in a shroud. He passed away Sunday, we waked him on Tuesday, and had the funeral immediately following the wake that same afternoon. It was a very rough three days! Normally, under Catholicism, it's a week or more. I was a mess; a complete train wreck. I completely lost it, bawling my eyes out when DBAG1 came to the wake, and stood in line waiting to hug me and pay her respects. I had not seen or spoken to her since all that had happened with LL1. I was grateful that she came, but all my emotions came pouring out; she had betrayed me, and on this day I was extremely vulnerable and emotional. Several of my dad's patients and employees attended his wake. When paying their respects, they told me how proud my dad was of me, and how he would brag about me and tell them how much he loved me. I never knew any of this; my dad never told me these things. Two times in my life my dad told me he loved me by age 23--only two times. Parents, tell your kids you love them, often! Please compliment and praise your children regularly. It does make a big difference in their lives. If you can't say it, write them a card or a note saying it. My mom did both and often.

We waked my dad on Tuesday that week and went straight to the cemetery for the funeral that same day. There are special plots for Muslims. While we were at his plot, everyone stayed to watch the casket going into the ground while the men threw dirt on it. My best friend's mom, who is Jewish, grabbed some dirt and threw it on his casket. Then I went up and started throwing dirt on too. After all, he was my father. The Muslim priest came right up to me and told me I could not do that since I was a female. I thought, "Who the hell are you to tell me I can't do this? It's my dad! It's his funeral!" I was bawling my eyes out. I am not a Muslim; I am a Catholic. We paid a substantial amount of money to wake him and pay for all of this. I did not listen to the Muslim priest and kept throwing the dirt. More females joined me.

My brother went back home to the west coast at the end of that week, so it was LL3 and I cleaning my dad's place. My mom did help some. I love my mom dearly, and I know that she too was grieving; however, she had asked for money to help us in cleaning his home and working on his estate. I know she had just gone through a divorce and having been married for thirty years she received half of his estate, so I didn't understand why she was asking for money. It was rather upsetting to me at the time. Death does funny things to people; families often fight over money and responsibilities. This was just a bad time for all this. When there is a death, some take advantage of how vulnerable you are. A pastor friend of my mom was a complete jerk to me regarding the sale of my father's car. I can't remember specifics today, but I know I should have told him to forget it. That's how mean he was to me. My mom did not stand up to him either. I was very upset. I remember having to call upstairs to LL3 to come down from my dad's condo and finish the transaction with my mom's pastor friend because I was too upset with the way he spoke to me. What is it with these priests and pastors? Seriously!

We shipped my brother a truck full of furniture from Chicago to the west coast. I took a few things from the house, like paintings and other odds and ends. Six months following my father's death, I became aware that something wasn't quite right. I was super depressed; I did not care about work, or anything. I only cared about me, and I became super selfish which I later found out is quite common after losing a loved one. My dad's best friend referred me to a psychiatrist; they prescribe meds. I knew I didn't need meds. I needed to speak and get my emotions out in the open. I did seek help with a counselor for a few years following my dad's death. This did help. After my dad died, I started taking interest in another guy at work. LL3 did not want to break up, so I started dating two guys at the same time. I had never dated two guys at the same time and I do not recommend it either! My dating this other guy did not last long; his true colors came out pretty quickly and I was done with him, plus I was lost from my father's death, and from my childhood wounds. LL3 and I were still together, but I treated him like crap. I put my friends and going out to the night clubs first. I was young and dumb. I went on vacation to Acapulco with girlfriends, and of course, we met some cute, fun boys. Nothing happened, but I did take a liking to a guy I met from NYC, and we kept in contact via email. LL3 had somehow come across my email, so I was busted. A few days later, I broke it off with LL3. At the time, I remember thinking that our relationship was too much work. Later on in my life, I realized that all relationships are hard work and that this was normal; no relationship is easy. If I were happy with myself, I wouldn't have been looking on the other side of the fence. I would not change anything today though. I do not want LL3 back. I just realize how horrible I was to him and how much I hurt him. Isn't that the way it goes for so many of us? We don't appreciate what we have in front of us until it's gone. LL3 was so loving and respectful; he treated me like gold and made me a priority, so for that I thank him. I did apologize to him later on. My actions toward him were due to all that was going on in my life, how immature I was at the time, and even my past relationship experiences, including my relationship with my father. I was not happy, and I was searching for it outside instead of turning inside for it. Happiness is an inside job, so I was wrong, so wrong in my actions. LL3 had made friends within my circle of male and female friends, so we remained friends following our breakup. Yes, it was awkward and difficult at first. After three months of being single which really was not a long time, I started dating LL4, who in my opinion was my AH-HA moment in life.

Life Lesson #4 aka LL4, My AH-HA Moment

Be with someone who knows exactly what they've got when they have you--Not someone who will realize it when they've lost you.

I met LL4 three months after the break up with LL3. We met through a girlfriend we both knew at Bally Total Fitness, where we worked at the time. I went out with my girlfriend to a bar, and we ran into LL4. We hung out that night and ended up hitting it off. Rewind a second: LL4 had actually bought the same girlfriend and me shots awhile back at a bar when I was dating LL3. Nothing happened; I just took the shot. I also would see him working out at the gym, and he would always stare at me in an angry, sort of creepy way. He would never smile at me, so I had no clue he had a crush on me. We both had to work a grand opening at Bally Total Fitness in Naperville in early June. I was part of the performance team, and he was part of the management team. He asked me to go out to a bar in the city, so it wasn't a dinner date. We hung out every day for a good week. He had asked me to go to his best friend's graduation party, so I met him there. He, of course, was bragging about me to all of his friends, telling them that I used to cheer for The Bulls (story of my life. More often than not, it's not a good thing; this I will explain later). When we left the party, we headed back to my place, and I had to carry him up the stairs since he was so drunk. We went out the next morning for breakfast; we did this a lot. This was a different time in my life. I was 26. I worked out 5-6 times a week, but I also went out every weekend, drank like a fish, and ate whatever I wanted.

After that first week, he spent a lot of time hanging out with his buddies. He was 22 and had just graduated college, so he was in that mode...so I thought.

About a month passed and I asked him what was going on between us, especially since other guys were asking me out. I did not want to date them; I wanted to date only LL4. He said, "Let's go out to lunch." He never really gave me an answer of "yes, we are dating exclusively," or "I'd like for you to be my girlfriend," but from that point forward we did date exclusively. He took me to Miami a few months later and told me this was the longest he had dated a girl. At that point, we had been dating five months. LL4 had never been in a long-term relationship. The beginning of our relationship revolved around going out and drinking. It was very hard to always be out and about in the scene due to my past relationships. I had a very hard time trusting him because I had been cheated on so many times in the past which was my bad; I never gave him the benefit of the doubt. Also, when he interacted with my girlfriends or other girls in general, he often gave them more attention than he gave me. I think a lot of men do this. Or are we women sensitive to this? We argued a lot, especially when drinking. Alcohol escalates things. For example, there was a night we were in the city at a bar, and I was holding his hand. While I was holding his hand, he attempted to kiss another brunette girl. I, of course, stopped him, and asked, "What are you doing?" He responded by saying he thought it was me because he was so drunk. She looked somewhat like me, dark hair and eyes, but it was definitely not me! I was holding his hand and holding him up at the same time.

Our families would travel together for my fitness competitions when I would compete on the West Coast. His mother, aunt, uncle, and paternal grandmother would fly out with my mom and my brother to watch me compete and get together as a family. His family loved attending my competitions, traveling for them, and visiting on holidays and birthdays. He often complained about my passion for fitness, performing, and competing though. LL4 moved in with me early on in our relationship, although he still lived at home. He was working at Bally Total Fitness in sales then. A few months later he switched to investment real estate and did extremely well. He was working under a senior partner when something happened. Things were not going his way, and he had to go at investment real estate alone, which he didn't want. Now, I personally would have just pushed through it. He ended up quitting and did not work for two years. For the first five years of our relationship, I was the bread winner. During those two years, he looked for a job but wasn't sure what he wanted to do. He had played hockey in college, but due to a shoulder injury could no longer play. He was a Wisconsin alumnus. When he was living with me (I was renting at the time), he helped pay for a cleaning service, which was his uncle's business. Once he lost his job, he was not paying for anything. When I discovered he was not going to be able to pay for the cleaners, I told him he needed to clean our place. He did not like this at all; he was lazy when it came to domestic stuff. Maybe it was the Leo in him!

When LL4 and I first started dating, we would talk on the phone daily. This was in 1999 long before texting was the norm. We got to know one another over time, but had sex early on in the relationship. If sex comes before a friendship or a foundation is built, it's harder to see the red flags and make the right choices. We women (and men too) use our heart instead of our head in situations where we need to just walk away. We get too emotionally attached because of the sex. Plus, many women don't have fathers who show them how a man should treat a woman. I didn't. Men should be with us to affirm us, not to "get something" from us. My parents were not a healthy example of what a healthy relationship should be. My family was not good at communicating, talking about emotions, or apologizing. I grew up and did much of the same in my twenties and early thirties.

As adults, it is hard to say no to sex. I don't think I need to explain that one as I am sure many would agree, even those who are big in their faith. LL4 started a huge argument with me in our second year of dating. We were out at a birthday dinner for his mom and me, since we both have November birthdays. He got into it with me because my mom was super late for this dinner, and he then said he wanted to break up. My mom was known for being late. It didn't matter who the event was for or where the event was, she was usually late--something we all accepted about her. She was a sweet, nonjudgmental women who would do anything for anyone. She was always kind and loving to LL4. After arguing back and forth awhile, he finally realized that he was being an idiot. I couldn't control my mom, she was not hurting him, and in the scheme of things, her tardiness wasn't something to complain about.

Since my dad's death, a lot of things did not stress me out as they would many people. I learned to "not sweat the small stuff" in my twenties and continue to even now in my forties. In 2003, when I turned 30, my mom had a surprise party for me at the house I had just bought, my first home. I had been working at Nordstrom since 1993 and I left in 2000. I worked in their sales promotional office as an intern my senior year of college. After graduation, I started in sales in Brass Plum, and then I transferred to The Concierge for a new store opening; they oversaw special events at that time. I was later promoted to the position of special event coordinator, which was an awesome position--right up my alley since I love to plan events. Nordstrom started to cut their budget and combined customer service with The Concierge, so I then was promoted to assistant customer service manager for the store. By this time, I had been employed there seven years. I was burned out. I did not have a life, especially during the major holidays. I worked every weekend until 11 pm or midnight, and I did not have any set days off. I also needed more money. I was not happy with my job anymore. It's always better to have a job while looking for a second job, so I stayed for another seven months until a better opportunity was presented to me. During that time, LL4 was there for me to vent regarding this situation. I told my boss I needed to cut back on my hours so I could look for a job and interview outside the company since she could not pay me more, or give me better hours or set days off. I found out she was not giving me a good report when I interviewed internally with other managers who had Monday through Friday, 9 am- 5 pm positions open. Not cool! She could fall in line as a douche bag.

She was upset I was leaving the department and even tried brainwashing me into believing I would not find a better job. Either way, it all worked out in my best interest as I was hired by Claire's corporate buying offices to work Monday through Friday, 8 am-5 pm with weekends off unless traveling for a few trade shows throughout the year. Ironically, after my third day working for Claire's, I received a call from Human Resources at the Oakbrook Nordstrom location offering me a management position. The GM at the Woodfield location also had offered me an assistant manager position on the selling floor to eventually work my way up to buyer. I did not accept either offer. It felt great to know others saw my value even though my direct boss didn't. This experience taught me that when people leave, they need to do what is best for them. My boss at that time held a grudge with me for being honest that I was unhappy and needed more. As a manager, one main job is to help your employees/ staff grow and move up the ladder in the company, even if that means losing a valuable employee. It's too bad. We were close friends too but that situation ended our friendship.

Every job except my first one out of college I got because of my networking or "friend working" skills. I am sure many of you get me on this. It's who you know as they know your work ethic and what you are capable of. At Claire's, I had my own office and had someone under me that I managed. I worked for them from 2000 to 2003. I loved this job and the people I worked with. I had so much fun with product development and being creative with girly stuff. LL4 had started working for his uncle's HVAC company in about 2002 (that's heating and air conditioning). He worked in sales for them part time about 15 hours a week. He dictated his own hours and would sleep in most weekdays. He spent a lot of time watching TV, reading, and on the computer. I bought my first house that year and at that time, he was not earning much money, so he wasn't paying the bills. So, I got a roommate to help pay rent. He did not like that, but he really had no say since he was not contributing to rent and did not own my house. However, when I look back, this was something I should have communicated to him but I didn't know better to include him and do that. She was the only roommate I lived with other than my roommate in college. She was an acquaintance at the time and over the next few years, we became close friends. Most girls are divas. I like my privacy and I didn't want anyone going into my room taking my clothes. She was very respectful of our space and my belongings, as was I in regards to her space and belongings. I bought a two bedroom, two bath house with a living room, kitchen, den, dining room, and attached garage. We had a lot of room, so it was the perfect size, plus it was about ten minutes from my work. After about a year, LL4 was able to contribute to paying rent and other household expenses.

I need to interject with my DBAG4 story here. She and I met back in 2001 and trained together a few nights a week. We also traveled to competitions together. In 2002, she competed and placed Top 20, which meant performing at finals and being published in *Oxygen* magazine. I competed as well, and did not make the Top 20 that year. There were usually around 80- 100 competitors, so the remaining athletes who did not make the Top 20 were asked to help those who did get dressed backstage, since it was a time crunched show. Not only did I help DBAG4, we also went out and celebrated that night at the clubs in Miami. In summer of 2003, I ended up making the Top 20, and she did not. DBAG4 was nowhere to be found when I needed help backstage getting dressed and such. She also was no-where to be found when out celebrating that night. I never even received a con-gratulations from her. LL4 was with me at this competition, and he knew how hurt I was that she was not there for me like I had been for her. He actually told her off to her face at the club that night, which didn't make matters any better. Either way, we never spoke again after that. It was quite sad to see how a good friend, so I thought, could not be happy for me and my success like I was for her.

Back to LL4; my mom had a surprise 30th birthday party for me at my new place. She even bought me new bedroom furniture as a gift. LL4 and I then got engaged in mid-2003. He wanted to propose in a hot-air balloon. Since the weather did not cooperate that day though, he was not able to do that. Instead he took me out to eat at our favorite steak house in Chicago. We were walking on the streets, it was a nice spring evening, and he just got down on one knee and proposed. I knew the engagement was coming since on a recent vacation in St. Thomas, we shopped for a diamond and a setting. We did find a beautiful setting and he found a diamond online. He did a lot of research on diamonds. He was very wise when it came to spending money, especially investing it. During our engagement, LL4 settled down a bit, meaning he was not out getting drunk and spending a ton of money as often as he had previously done. Claire's had a buy out for the department I worked in from a company on the West Coast called Worldwide Cosmetics. I ended up going with this buyout. My boss at the time went with the buyout as well except he moved from Florida to California. I worked from home and commuted back and forth from Chicago to North Hollywood, California. A few employees lost their jobs due to this buy out. I was grateful that I was able to continue in the same line of work.

I enjoyed working for Worldwide. I had a lot of flexibility working from home even though they kept me busy day and night. My days would not start until 9 or 10 am, and I would work on and off through the day until about 8 or 10 pm depending on various projects or if I needed to contact factories overseas. I would travel out to California for ten days at a time typically.

Interview with my boss Dino from Claire's and Worldwide Cosmetics:

I first met Nicole when I was President of a company called Sassy Doo! It was a division of Claire's stores. She was hired as a buyer. I saw so much potential in her. She stood out and she was a hard worker. We had a trip coming up to Minneapolis from Chicago. She was in casual clothes when traveling, so she asked to be excused to the ladies room to change into a more formal outfit, and when she came out it was like Cinderella had arrived. She was perfect, all in her red suit.

We went to Target (an account of ours at Claire's). While driving I told her I wanted her to make the presentation; she knew more about the product than I did. She was all over the place, trying to back out of it, but she really knew the product better than anyone. We got to where we needed to be and set up the product line. I then turned to her and told her the ball was in her court. I went to the back of the room and told her to look at me. She talked a little fast at first; I am sure it was just nerves. I gave her a small hand movement to slow down and she nailed it. She did a "perfect" delivery of the product. She smiled the whole time; she has a great smile. We got the order. On our way back to the airport, she told me she felt like a million dollars. I told her, "You always had this in you; you just needed a shot to prove it, and someone to help bring that out of you."

Ever since then we've been great friends. She is a great person who loves helping people and being there for them. Pardon my French but she has balls, too. Nicole is not afraid to speak her mind. She is opinionated, and it sets her apart. Another reason why I grew fond of her: she did not "yes" me to death. On a trip to Vegas one year, she was working a booth for me and someone asked her where her father was. Everyone thought she was my daughter. I got a kick out of it and ever since then I feel I became somewhat of a father figure to her, especially since her dad is deceased. I do see her as a daughter to this day, and I am very happy for her and all of her accomplishments.

After a year, Conair bought out the line I managed; they are based on the East Coast. Conair offered me a job as long as I moved out east to work for them. I did not want to move; I wanted to continue to work from home, especially since things did not work out for the line I managed with the California based company. Who's to say it won't be the case that I move out east and things don't work again? I started interviewing in the Chicagoland area, and I was offered a great paying job in my field, except it was about a 45- 60 minute commute one-way during non-rush hour. When I told Conair I had received this job offer, they immediately offered me a job with them working from home making $20K more with health benefits, 401K, and profit sharing. This was perfect! Everything worked out. I spent most of my time working from home and planning my wedding. Unfortunately, my boss at Conair did not put my brain to use while I was at home. She micromanaged but didn't know how to assign projects for me to do at home. My boss told me she would call or email projects and then forget about me. When I was out of sight, I was out of mind. Some may think this was great with my wedding planning, which it was, but when it came time to update my resume, I had nothing to add to it. When you accept a new job offer, it's typical that one walks away with new skills and responsibilities to add to their resume. That was not the case with this job/ boss. I would fly into LaGuardia Airport, then drive a rental car to Conair which is based in Stamford, CT. I traveled there once a month or every other month for one to two weeks at a time and would stay in their company home. When in town at corporate, I was kept busy and quite productive my entire stay.

During my relationship with LL4, I often would hang out with my male and female friends in the area. We would watch *The Sopranos* on Sundays, celebrate birthday dinners out, hit the clubs in the city, and the list goes on, but LL4 would rarely go to anything with me. I would always invite him to come along but he usually would sit home on the couch watching TV, playing video games, or nursing his hangovers. In the ten years we were together, I can count on one hand how many times he worked out at the gym with me, yet we met at Bally Total Fitness. I literally would have to cry to get him to do anything with me for that matter. It finally got to the point where I stopped asking. I wanted someone to be with me because they wanted to, not because I had to beg them to be. As I reflect back now, I see the example my parents gave me. They did not spend much time together. My dad put his career first (which so many people do, especially if they are unhappy in their marriage or with themselves) and my mom was very independent. Instead of working to resolve reoccurring issues with my father, she too turned outward. After raising my brother and me, she returned to work when I was about 12 years of age. She started her own business and later worked part-time in nursing. So in my marriage, I accepted us not always hanging out and doing things together as "normal," if that makes sense. Our family of origin has such an impact on us, not just in our own personal development but even in the relationships we build in our adult years. I learned many unhealthy behaviors from my parents which is not to say they were bad people but just bad examples as far as marriage. Isn't this the case for most families today? It is sad. We need schools for marriage and parenting. I saw how my parents would ignore one another for months! I too did the same if upset with LL4. I did not have the tools to resolve problems in our marriage and neither did my parents. I watched my mother "put up" with how my father mistreated her. She was "comfortable" as was I; too afraid to speak up and share my feelings. I did not know how to set boundaries.

Back to LL4; planning our wedding was awesome, especially since I had a background in event planning. Our wedding was amazing and I know those who attended would agree. The venue was The Adler Planetarium on Lake Michigan in downtown Chicago; what a spectacular view and incredible backdrop for wedding pictures. My wedding gift to LL4 was singing him a song at our wedding reception. I surprised him. He often would lose things I gave him, like the wedding ring I bought him even. That's just one of many examples. I figured he couldn't lose a song and that would be a memory he would keep for a lifetime. I have danced my entire life but singing I stink at. I took lessons every week for about a year prior to our wedding. He had no clue about these lessons; I am good at surprises. When I sang he actually started to cry...tears of joy. I picked "Be My Little Baby" by The Ronettes. My bridesmaids were my backup singers and dancers. It was so much fun and a surprise for all guests attending.

At this point, LL4 was making good money, so we split the cost of the wedding. We had 300 people at our wedding and of that count, 100 friends of mine. It was a huge wedding. Since I have held several leadership positions and worked in product development, I like to do things my way. I can be vocal and a bit of a control freak at times, or I guess just very particular about the way I want things. If you are just like me, thumbs up! I like being unique and creative. At the head table, I had the most important people sit with us; we included my mom, my brother, LL4's mom and grandparents, along with the best man, matron of honor and their spouses. I really do not like attending weddings where I don't get to sit with my date. I seated our wedding party with their dates at two tables next to us. I made picture boards of us over the years for guests to look at during cocktail hour and following dinner and we also hired a barbershop quartet for the cocktail hour. My mom gave me this hook-up. The venue even accommodated my seating requests; some tables had 11 guests, others 9. We also booked The W Bar for an after-party for guests following the wedding. This was great because we were able to invite other friends who we did not invite to our wedding but still wanted to include on our special day. Our wedding day and night really was perfect.

We left for Australia for our honeymoon two days following. We ate so much crap on this trip that it was like Christmas, eight days in a row. When we got back home, I did my very first detox. I was bloated and felt yucky from all the food we had eaten. I did a three day cleanse of juicing vegetables with a clay detox. I followed a plan from Partners in Wellness in Chicago. A friend had turned me on to Alyce, her detox website, and her business. People would be amazed at the amount of energy and good stuff you get from homemade vegetable broth. I was on liquids, as well as vegetable and fruit juices for three days. When people do this type of cleanse or detox it is meant to give your digestive system a rest and eliminate the toxins built up. Hence no working out; you need to replenish after working out and on this type of detox the liquids are not enough. I also did an organic coffee enema. Say what? I know it sounds crazy. It was hard; I had to have my husband help me with that. I did this for three days. I could not do it for the seven that the plan suggested because I really was craving meat. When I look back now, I probably should have pushed through to the seven days at that point. After three days of this detox I felt fabulous. I had so much energy and lost my bloat. This was the start of me finally taking my nutrition and health to the next level.

How many angels do you have in your life; you know, the ones who introduce you to a certain person or educate you on certain topics which end up changing your life? Often, the first time you hear about something it can go in one ear and out the other. It was not until about the third time I heard about detoxing, and that I needed one, that I did it. When I taught resistance training classes at Bally Total Fitness, a member named Donna who took my class regularly said I was toxic since I was always sick and that I needed a detox. On the outside I looked healthy but on the inside, my body was dying. I have to thank her. She really opened my eyes to a major lifestyle change. She too had been diagnosed with Candida and had pretty much been through a lot of what I had been through as far as my health history. She was my cheerleader during my detox with my integrative chiropractor. Another reason I selected the quote I have at the beginning of the book on suffering and how we all go through it: to help others with their suffering.

About a month after LL4 and I married, we went to marital counseling per my request. Being in sales, my husband could work whatever hours he wanted. One of my husband's good friends that he went to high school with was going through a divorce, so he would go out with this friend on weeknights to bars until the wee hours of the morning. He also got a DUI during that time and came home wasted whenever out with friends. He came home late one night and woke me up (which was a common occurrence). At that time, I had 5:30 am personal training clients. I expressed to him that this was a recurring problem, and that I would not tolerate it anymore. I told him we needed to go to marital counseling. There were many other issues between us besides this, but this was the icing on the cake. Surprisingly, he agreed.

When we arrived at our counselor's office, we filled out the forms to start couple's counseling. After this, she asked to meet with each of us individually first before meeting as a couple. When she sat down with me, I told her that my husband was an alcoholic. The first thing she said to me was that if he was truly an alcoholic, she could not save our marriage because he would live in denial. People think the definition of an alcoholic is being sloppy drunk all the time. This is not the case. LL4 would typically be on drink number three while I was still on drink number one. He would black out often, not remembering what had happened the previous night. LL4 would always tell me I was no fun because I would not drink or I would not drink as much as he did. Everyone else in my life told me I was fun and uplifting to be around, especially when sober. He often told me I had a drinking problem and would get angry if I said he had a problem. One day I mentioned his drinking in therapy to Glory, our counselor. When we got home that night, he told me to never bring up his drinking again when in therapy. I told him OK and never did. He obviously did not want to go there or admit anything. With Glory's expertise I focused on me and my issues, which is really the whole point of counseling. The first year of counseling I worked on me--the biggest misconception couples have about marital counseling is that they think it's about trying to change one another instead of learning and better understanding one another. You learn yourself, your partner, what works, what doesn't, healthy tools to communicate and fight fairly, and how to set boundaries. It is not meant to change your partner; remember we can only change and better ourselves if we want to.

"When it's difficult or destructive we want to work harder. God calls us to honor our spouse the same as honoring our parents." - Tony Evans

One of my biggest issues was trust, especially since I had been cheated on twice in the past. I blamed LL4 for not treating me the way he "should have." He had never dated long-term before and with his mom raising him herself, I'm not sure if he ever had any good examples of how a man should treat a woman. He often disrespected me in public and in private, and didn't make a habit of making me feel special. It was around this time that LL1 apologized to me. His apology, along with the self-awareness and tools I gained in counseling helped me regain my trust in others, especially LL4. Or a better way of putting it, counseling taught me how not to react and how to live in the present moment.

Do you have the tools or know the steps to get through your relationships? If not, seek help through books, YouTube, counseling, or even your church.

Once issues I needed to work on were pointed out in therapy, LL4 would then ask me if I would work on them, which I did. To this day I still am working on me. I learned to listen to my partner's needs and more importantly, I learned to take a step back and pause versus reacting in the heat of the moment. I am not perfect and still at times react today, but I have come a long way from where I used to be. With therapy, I learned not to engage in an argument; it takes two to have a fight and escalate things, meaning, it can get out of control to the point where one says and does things one really regrets. In learning to step back, listen and be more present, I did not revert back to that hurt little girl from the past.

After the first year, LL4 was not working on himself, at least not his anger or his drinking. It was just like Glory said in our first meeting. I was working on myself and our relationship, but he wasn't; he was living in denial. I was admitting my issues and working with Glory on how to unlearn unhealthy behaviors and patterns and change myself for the better, because I wanted to. LL4 had put in effort when it came to dialogues and a few other things. Dialogues are a tool Glory gave us to communicate feelings when upset with your partner or yourself--a healthier, safer way to express emotions with your partner. However, he was not admitting to an anger problem or how he handled his temper in various situations. When you're married, it's a tug a war; a lot of back and forth. One person is working and the other is not. It is quite a task to get both parties to put in the work needed at the same exact time. You need healthy tools and healthy ways to fix problems so they don't keep popping up. I had a lot of unhealthy tools in my relationship toolbox, as did he. I often shut down on him. If I was upset or hurt, I would not talk to him. I am not blaming this on my dad, but this is what I learned in my family of origin. My dad would not speak to my mother for weeks, months, and even a year at a time. As I mentioned with LL2, my father ignored me and cut me out of his life for a good two years. As I look back now, I was extremely afraid of my father and telling him any of my feelings because they just didn't seem to matter. I was the same way with my husband. I didn't know how to communicate my feelings in a healthy manner. I was afraid of his reaction; that he just didn't care about me or about my feelings. Even though we learned what tools to use to better communicate in our marriage, we still were having problems. Alcohol was first in his life. I was not.

If you're in a destructive relationship you need to own your problem. Not fix their problem.

As our relationship continued, he would pour himself into drinking, and I would pour myself into my work or competing.

You can have a great marriage and a shitty career but still be happy. You can have a shitty marriage and a great career and still be miserable.

Isn't that what most people do? Turn to their work as an outlet instead of inward to their spouse to repair and build a stronger relationship. I am sure many of you are guilty of turning outward during difficult times versus inward to your spouse. It is much easier.

When your career, hobby or unhealthy habits get in the way of loving your spouse or the betterment of your relationship you need to make changes in your career, hobby or habits. If you have to leave home so much, you've failed. Stop letting the outside world dictate the world inside. Praise more of your spouse to them, to your children, and to your peers.

Many people, even people who didn't know me, assumed that I was too busy for LL4 and that I was never there for him. Assumptions are the termites of any relationship. I don't get pissed off often, but when people talk smack behind my back or to my face without ever having a conversation with me asking me any of these questions, yes I get quite upset! I was never too busy for him. I wanted him in my life and by my side for everything. I included him all the time. He would tell me "no" and sit on the couch watching TV or playing video games. He would go out with his friends and never include me. You finally get to a point where you stop asking and you start drifting further apart. I grew up watching my parents do the same. I just accepted this and remained comfortable. I did not know what to do. I was too scared to just walk away. People, men and women, often tell me they enjoy my company, and that they enjoy being around me. My husband did not want to be in my life, and that hurt. We met at Bally Total Fitness, a gym where we both worked, yet he only worked out with me three, maybe four times in ten years. Again, I learned to accept being apart as a couple from my parents' relationship. I learned that not being together was normal, or so I thought. When we had family parties to attend, on his side especially, he would often go with his mom or we would meet because many times he would tell me last minute and I already would have plans, so I would meet up with them later. We rarely went to family parties on his side together. All the other couples on his side of the family would come together, even if they arrived late and they would leave together.

When our one year anniversary came around, his mother called and said she wanted to celebrate by taking us out to dinner. LL4 did not set this up; his mom did. It would have meant the world to have LL4 plan our first wedding anniversary celebration, not his mother. She could have planned our ten year anniversary (had we been married that long) and that would have been fantastic. The weekend of our anniversary, a few of his buddies were in town. He went out with them downtown and stayed the night in a hotel. He never included me in this outing either. When he came back from the city, we did dinner out with both our moms. I was so upset! He never even called me that morning! Nothing! Not a word from him about our anniversary. He did later tell me that he had left flowers on my car. I had worked out that afternoon at the gym but I never received any flowers, so I thought he had lied. Come to find out, he put flowers on the wrong car. My boss told me later that week that another member brought the flowers to him since the card had my name on it. That day was very hard for me. I remember I broke down in my car; this was my first real breakdown. I was bawling my eyes out, crying uncontrollably. I called my counselor, and she calmed me down and asked me a few questions. Turns out this anniversary situation was bringing back painful childhood memories of when my dad would abandon and neglect me. I have major abandonment and neglect issues which I am not ashamed to share. Many of us do, but never really put a finger on it. I married my dad. My father was not an alcoholic, but my Brother Anonymous called my dad a dry drunk. Dads need to "date" their daughters to teach them how a man should treat them. My father never "dated" me. He would come and go and buy me things but he was not a constant presence in my life. I couldn't count on him to be there when it mattered most nor did we have an emotional connection, one with open honest communication. I've had many years to reflect on this. In my thirties, I was able to put myself in my father's shoes knowing his traumatic childhood and his upbringing. So many of us repeat both the good and bad examples laid out for us by our parents, and we also tend to pick partners similar to them.

I was still competing in fitness after we married. It was a positive outlet for me. I made so many friends from all around the world, got into fitness modeling, and I was still performing on stage, something I was truly passionate about. Plus, it kept me busy; it kept me away from my marriage and the repair work I was avoiding. This brings me to DBAG5, a Ms. Fitness USA competitor. The year prior when I competed in this federation for the first time, I placed ninth in the USA on my own merit and won $1000 in home gym equipment. Plus, my performance was aired on Fox Sports Net. My second year competing in this federation, I came back with the same physique if not better and I nailed my fitness routine performance as well as my speech in the evening gown round. It's typical for competitors in this federation to place higher with each passing year. During the long weekend in Las Vegas, we had a lot of time to interact and hang with the other female competitors. One female competitor bullied me quite a bit throughout the weekend. Others even witnessed it, and a few stuck up for me. Again, it was another girl I never did anything to. At the end of the event when they announced placings and prizes, I did not make the Top 15. I was very upset. I left crying. LL4 and another good guy friend of mine were there to take me out that night and listen to me sob over not placing. Really, there are bigger problems in the world, and here I was bawling over a competition placing. Once I got home, I emailed the judges asking for feedback and one responded. He said that my behavior off-stage needed to be corrected. I was like, huh? What did I do and how does what I do off stage affect my placing on stage? He said, my attitude. I was still clueless. I responded with, "Well if that is the case then you need to look at your Top 5 this year" (the girl who bullied me placed second). I did not even mention her name but the judge did respond saying he knew who I was referring to and even mentioned her name in his email to me. He said he had supposedly spoken to her about her attitude but he also happened to be her coach. So, it was OK for her to have an attitude off-stage and place second but not me (even though I did not have an attitude, it was a lie as to why I didn't place).

Fast forward two years later to 2007. I decided to compete in a local show so my family and my husband's family could watch. Again, they loved attending and supporting me at fitness competitions. I emailed the promoter who happened to be the head judge of Ms. Fitness USA. He was so happy I emailed him that I was competing again. This was a different judge than the one I had emailed before. He told me that he had gotten into an argument with the other judge regarding my placing the year prior. He said I should have placed much higher that year, and that my physique and performance were perfect. Well, that made my day and my year! After competing in the local show, I won which qualified me for Ms. Fitness USA again and I decided to compete that year. I wind up seeing DBAG5 there; she was competing. I ended up placing seventh at USAs, higher than DBAG5. It is funny how the tables turn and karma does its job. The best part of this story is that I did not give up because of a douchebag! While on stage, I was scouted by a producer who shoots fitness infomercials and commercials in California. LL4 did not attend the competition with me that year so after competing, I was walking back to my hotel room alone, passing through the casino and heard some random man shouting at me. The man was this producer. He introduced himself, and told me he was shooting soon and loved my physique. He asked for my business card and said he would be in touch. About a week later, I received a call from him asking my rates and telling me about the modeling job in California. He was 100% legit. I was flown out several times to San Diego to shoot between 2007 and 2010. To think I almost did not talk to this stranger, and I almost did not return to compete again in Ms. Fitness USA that year. I am so glad I did. The infomercials and commercials aired nationwide and in Canada over the years. It was pretty cool to get calls from people saying they saw me on TV and then to finally see myself as well. My mom would wake up at 6 am for months to watch me on TV in Chicago.

Since LL4 more often than not complained while at these events, I decided that it was best that he stay home when I traveled to competitions. When traveling to California and Miami, he only wanted to go out and party. Competing is a selfish sport. It's all about "me" and "I", not about "we" and "us". Heck, who wouldn't want to go out on the town when traveling? However, being that my lifestyle and hobby were "healthy" I needed my beauty rest for the event and scheduled photo shoots. If we went out on the town, it was usually the last night there. The party life style was getting old, at least for me. He was bringing me down. I needed people in my life that would lift me up or support me, and at this point, it wasn't my husband. For example, I encouraged him in many ways to do so much more with his life outside of his sales job. Even though he was making six figures and dictated his own schedule, he wasn't quite satisfied with his job. He did share this with me. He did some volunteer work which was great and we sometimes would do this together, assuming we were getting along at the time of the event. I signed him up for MMA classes in 2007 as Christmas present. He ended up really enjoying this and continued. He made several friends with this new hobby, and even started his own clothing and event business around MMA. It's funny because as I was exiting the fashion/ retail/ special event industries, he was just starting. In August of 2008, I was blindsided. My husband left home for two weeks and did not want to be contacted during that time. He was at his grandparents' house. When we finally talked, he explained how upset he was that I was always putting fitness and competing first. I agreed and explained that his alcohol and nights out with friends came before me and how upset I was. I told him that both of us needed to work at putting "us" before anything else. We needed to make us and our relationship a priority. He came home after our discussion. Ironically, at this same time, I had an appointment with my integrative doctor who performed an MSA (Meridian Stress Assessment). For the first time, my heart showed up in the red zone. My heart was stressed and hurting from the physical absence of my husband.

Does your partner support your goals in life? "Your partner would ideally lift you into your highest life purpose." - Jason Nelson

Con-Artist #1

In 2008, I met the devil and didn't know it. Have you ever been on Myspace? A guy messaged me on it saying he had seen me on TV, in magazines, and on the competition scene. He said he too had been published in magazines, and that we should do a shoot together and get our work published. He listed his number to contact him to set up a photo shoot. I did not respond. About two months later, I got another message from him. He wrote the same message again. I finally called the guy; he lived in Chicago at the time. We ended up discussing setting up a photo shoot in the near future. I then ran into him in early October at a competition. He actually competed in bodybuilding for the first time at this show. I did not see him on stage; he approached me at a booth where I was working at the event. Con-Artist #1 (CA1) is also a major life lesson, but I prefer to call him a slimeball too. My story is about to get real juicy.

During this same time, my husband and I had just bought our first home together. We went shopping a lot to get furniture and other items needed for our new home. At this point, LL4 was very mean and emotionally abusive to me so he was totally miserable to be around. We'd go out with my friends to celebrate birthdays or weddings, and LL4 would often bring me to tears in the car ride there or home. My therapist suggested that next time this happened, ask him to stop the car and just get out and walk home. I never did do this. I was too scared; how would I get home or into the house if I didn't have a house key, and so on? However, it would have been a good boundary to set to let him know I would not tolerate his unhealthy behavior and abuse. We had a move-in date of a Friday in late November but things were still the same. At night LL4 would be on the computer, watching TV, playing XBOX, or out at the bars with friends. I would be on the phone talking to CA1 though. I talked with him every night for a good two months and we got pretty close. My husband never went to bed with me; he usually would go to bed after midnight. CA1 and I grew a strong emotional connection with one another because he gave me what I needed. He totally filled a void that I wasn't getting from my husband.

The weekend we moved in to the new house, LL4 asked one of his MMA buddies to come help hang pictures and a few other things that he did not know how to do. Since his father was never in his life, he never had a man teach him how to be domesticated or handy around the house. He was definitely very intelligent regarding real estate and finances, but not household duties, which is OK because I don't know how to do-it-all either; just trying to make a point in my story. That night after they finished hanging pictures, he told me they were going to the bar. I was livid! We had just bought a $500,000 home and the first weekend in it, instead of unpacking together, he was going to go to the bar with a friend? To top it off he didn't even invite me to come with. At this point, I was fuming. I told him he hadn't even invited me to go along. He said, "Oh, you can come with." I said, "No thanks. I would rather you want to include me versus me begging or forcing you to include me." The following week in therapy, I brought up all this stuff that had been going on. My therapist asked LL4 if he thought he had an anger problem. He said, "Hmmm, I kind of have an anger problem." That was the first time in 3.5 years that he admitted he had an anger problem, "kind of"! He admitted to being stressed out since this was his first home purchase, that he was scared, and that he had taken his anger out on me, so my therapist wanted to see us separately going forward. I had only wished that he had shared with me that the house was stressing him out. That was the relationship I was seeking: one where we could communicate our feelings regarding almost anything versus reacting and taking things out on each another. I often was his punching bag. I know this is the case in many relationships, and I too have been guilty of the same. It's too bad we are never taught how to express our emotions in a healthy manner, both men and women. Maybe some are lucky in their family of origin or through counseling classes or workshops, but most of us never learn a healthy, safe way to tell someone how we feel. Furthermore, most misinterpret shared feelings as personal attacks.

You can live in the same home and not have oneness. We had no oneness, and it sucked!

We met separately with the counselor up until Christmas. After Christmas we were vacationing in California for a few days. In the last session I had with Glory before heading on vacation, she asked, "Nicole, if you're that unhappy, why don't you get out of your marriage?" The session ended right there; she had another appointment following mine, and I had another appointment to run to myself. I was like, oh boy, now what? I used to be the bread winner, but now he was. We had just bought a house. How would I survive if I moved out? It was the holidays. We were going on vacation. It just wasn't a good time. Really, there never is a perfect time to end any relationship, is there? How could I file for divorce now? CA1 and I talked and texted while on vacation. While there, I had an appointment at a modeling agency. While I was driving back from the agency, my phone was not working. I thought I didn't have service since I was driving through the mountains. When I got back to the hotel, my husband surprised me with an iPhone. He turned off the phone I had, and activated the new one he bought. I was blown away and freaking out, thinking he was going to see that CA1 had been texting me. Thankfully, he didn't. We headed out to dinner later that night--not a bar, dinner mind you. LL4 still passed out in bed when we returned home from drinking a lot at dinner though. I did not drink that night.

I spent a good hour in the bathroom talking to CA1 on the phone that night. When we returned home to Chicago, CA1 and I made plans to meet up face-to-face, alone. At this point, we were intimate but had never had sex. On New Year's Eve, LL4 and I went to a Bulls game together and we came home early that night. I went to bed by myself. My husband and I did not even ring in the New Year together. He was downstairs while I was on the phone with CA1 who was in Miami celebrating the New Year. At the end of that first week of January, my husband came upstairs to our bathroom; he rarely came upstairs. I was in the bathroom and my cell phone rang. It was CA1. I answered and said, "I'll call you back later." I did not want to leave it ringing because LL4 would ask why I was not picking up the call. Since I hung up quickly on CA1, he texted me, "What's wrong baby?" My husband saw this text and he asked who it was. I said, "It's just a client" and he responded, "Really? I am sure your employer would consider that sexual harassment if a client was calling you baby." I was now freaking out and my heart was racing. I came clean and admitted I was having an emotional affair, but that we had never slept together.

"Sin is pleasurable for a season." - The Bible

"Before you judge me, make sure you're perfect." - Unknown

That night LL4 opened up to me like never before. He started asking me a lot of questions. We had been together nine years and for the first time he told me he was scared to have children. He would never talk about children. Every time relatives, friends, or I would bring it up, LL4 would change the subject. We rarely did anything with other couples. If we did, it was because we had a wedding or some special event. He told me he wanted to start doing everything as a couple; no more "me" or "I", it would be "we". I told him that I could not tolerate his drinking, and that I knew it was his first priority. I needed him to go to AA in order for me to stay in our marriage. He said he would not do that. I told him that there was no us if he couldn't go to AA. Alcohol was his mistress for our entire relationship; it came before me and us.

The next day, I called our marriage counselor and made an appointment that same day to see her. After I told her all that happened, she said, "Nicole I am glad you did something finally. I am not glad you had an affair, but I am glad you did something. I see it all the time with couples; every time the woman has an affair, the man can't change quickly enough." She said, "One of two things happen when women have affairs. They change; the man and they as a couple live happily ever after learning how to make each other a priority, or the women are done, and just want to wipe their hands clean and move on." LL4 went to therapy five times in that one week following the news of my having an affair! At the end of the week, I had to attend the wake of a friend's parent, and he wanted to go but I said no. For me, it was too late that he now wanted to be in my life. It took another man coming in to my life for him to appreciate me more? For the first time in our relationship, he admitted to and apologized for putting his drinking first in our relationship. He admitted to using it as an outlet. He admitted that this was why he did not want me to share in his life, and why he did not include me when out with his friends. He also told me he wanted to work on our relationship and stay married. Two people needing and wanting to work at their relationship at the same time is what a marriage is; it is something you have to work on every single day. More often than not, both partners aren't willing to work on their relationship at the same time. At this point, I wasn't expecting to stay in my marriage. I didn't expect my husband to want to stay married and work on us. I was confused, exhausted, and hurt.

I left home for three weeks in January of 2009. I cut off CA1 during that time too so I could be alone to make a decision and think clearly. I stayed at a close friend's house and a local hotel. I never told LL4 what hotel I was at. One morning I got a phone call from my husband. He was outside the hotel (he saw my car) and asked if he could come up and talk with me. He came up to my room, started talking and broke down crying. He told me he had talked with his uncle who owns the business he works for. His uncle is married with two children, so he reached out to him for advice (his real father was not in his life). He admitted that he never put me first or made us a priority. He said he wanted to do this going forward and he apologized again. He told me to take my time to gather my thoughts and to come back home when I was ready. He said that when I returned home, he wanted to know everything that had happened with this other guy. I shared my story with my mom and afterwards, she took me to see the movie *Eat Pray Love*. I recommend the movie or the book for anyone who is married or divorced.

As I was healing from my detox, I was not merely healing my body, but I was also healing emotionally. I had so much baggage from my deceased father and previous relationships that was weighing me down in the present moment. Both my integrative chiropractor and my marriage counselor helped me heal in many ways so I could move on in my life. Here I was, stuck between a rock and a hard place, saying God give me an answer. Do I stay in my marriage, for better or worse? I heard LL4 numerous times say that he was going to stop drinking only to start up again. It is so hard to be in a relationship when you're not first; it hurts so badly when you're being neglected. It's too painful, especially having been neglected by my father too. Those of you who have been in or currently are in relationships with addicts can relate. Therapy helped put things in perspective, and I was able to see the other side. Hurt people hurt other people, but don't always know it. I had been that hurt person hurting others until in marital counseling my unhealthy behaviors were brought to my attention and I made changes to unlearn them. I learned that when people react, it is about them. My reaction to LL4 would only escalate things between us. I learned to be more present, which helped when arguments came up. I also was more at peace with myself because I forgave my father without any apology even after he was gone. I accepted me and realized I was good enough, no matter what anyone in my past had told me. I learned that we cannot change anyone; they have to want to change themselves with the help of God. None of this was about me. I was trying to change my husband all along and, of course, he resisted. We women have a tendency to do that. He needed to want to change and better himself for himself. I have always wanted to do better and be a better person throughout my entire life. This is how you grow. Here I was trying so hard to change him and it was a complete fail. I was still so lost, not knowing which path to take.

I made a call to a guru. Remember how in *Eat, Pray Love*, Liz (Julia Roberts's character) went to visit a guru? The guru I contacted was an emotional intuitive based out of Texas. The call with her lasted an hour and all I told her was my first name. From that, she told me so many things that were happening in my life at that time and she told me about my future. I will never do this again. I never want to know my future, plus it goes against God's plan. I tried so hard to change and fight all the things she had told me would happen in my life that I didn't want to happen. The day after LL4 found out about my affair, I got the shingles, on my butt. How's that for karma? Here I am, a fitness/ health expert and bikini model who gets shingles-- on her ass! If you have had chicken pox which I did in my childhood, shingles comes on from emotional trauma or a suppressed immune system. The guru told me, "I am sensing a lot of heat." Now if you know anything about shingles, they are burning hot, and very painful. Again, she knew nothing about my situation or that I had the shingles; she only knew my name. I missed a day of work because of them, and had to resort to a prescription antiviral to stop it from regenerating for a few days since natural remedies did not help. She stated many other things about my current life as well, even about my health about which she was spot on. I was so afraid to tell LL4 the truth about how unhappy I was, and that I wanted to exit our marriage. I had had so many painful emotions trapped inside of me for so many years, and I was afraid of so many things. I was really lost, looking outside my marriage for happiness. The grass is not greener! I realized later, much later that the answer was inside of me, not another person.

My affair seemed innocent at first. Things weren't going well at home, and I was hungry for love and attention from one man. I needed to talk with my spouse instead; things needed to be said to LL4, not CA1. I opened up and turned my heart to someone else. I knew it was wrong.

I decided to come back home toward the end of January and work on our marriage. When I came home, we sat down to discuss all that had happened with "the other guy." I came clean and told LL4 we were emotionally and sexually intimate, but did not have sex, which was the truth. When he heard me say this, he broke the window treatment in our living room. Rightfully so. He then walked right up to me, got in my face and said these exact words to me: "I know why you did it. I was not there for you. I neglected you." How many of you reading this had an affair and your spouse found out? How many of you have heard this type of a response from your spouse? Not many, I am guessing. I commend LL4 for this. He took ownership, whereas most people would call the woman a slut or a whore, blaming her and more. He never would have owned up without the years of marital counseling. We both individually looked at ourselves and how we had contributed to the demise of our marriage, especially during that five days in a row of counseling he went to after he found out about my affair.

The best thing I got out of my marriage was LL4's apology, his acknowledgement of owning the problem, and his learning more about what I needed and how to ask for it. I say "best thing" as it helped me heal in many ways. You fall in and out of love over and over again. Look at the Clintons, for example. When you hit rock bottom and make a comeback that is when you hit the top because you know that nothing can break your marriage.

You never want anyone to know you have problems in your marriage. Marriage is emotional, physical and spiritual. You cannot pursue any of this alone. It has to be with intention that two people grow together, fully known as intimacy.

LL4 wrote me a heartfelt letter after my affair. Here are a few parts of it: "Going forward," he said, "no more 'I' or 'you' or 'me', it will always be 'we'." We would plan all things together going forward. We would be doing activities together. He said he would no longer drink alcohol. He would put me first above friends and family. He also said he would be more in tune with my concerns and feelings. He was ready to open up and be emotionally available. Partners often view their spouses as unapproachable and most relationships fail because of a lack of intimacy.

We had no intimacy. Think about it. Isn't it often times easier to go outside of your marriage (to friends, family, work, people of the opposite sex, hobbies, addictions, etc.) than it is to turn inward and work hard to communicate better with each other to grow stronger together? Isn't it just easier to stuff it under the rug and forget about it, burying it deep down inside of you where it harbors and builds up, eating you alive emotionally causing chronic health problems, ignoring your feelings until one day you explode like a bomb toward your partner or some other innocent bystander?

If married, always seek counsel from your spouse. Every relationship has problems, but if you can work through them, it makes the relationship stronger.

Most couples don't have the tools to fight fair. Don't we usually grow closer in times of conflict? We go to school to get an education and learn how to excel in the world and in business, but where do we learn to excel in our relationships? From our family of origin. Many of us come from dysfunctional families or broken homes. We learn from the examples our parents give or don't give us, they learn from their parents, and so on. It's not that our parents are bad people; they just do the best with what they learned. Marriage and parenting schools would greatly benefit everyone. I also think high schools and colleges should require classes on these two subjects. The world needs it! Oprah, I hope you're reading this. I didn't get married to have an affair; really, who does? I sinned and made a mistake, but was it really a mistake or a much needed life lesson to bring me where I am today? If I sin, it's because I want to. God doesn't keep our dresses down or our zippers up. Am I sounding like Carrie Bradshaw from *Sex and the City*? Ha!

It's quite sad that our marriage and dreams of living happily ever after-- all our hopes, wishes, and dreams-- came crumbing down. I am not a liar. I am an honest person. However, in this area of my life, I was so unhappy with myself that I became a liar and lied to my spouse. Growing up, I was always trying to please my father and win his approval. He often criticized me, telling me what he wanted me to do, and so forth. I was scared of him; scared to talk to him or share my feelings with him. This was the first relationship I ever had with a man, as it is with any girl (if her father is even present in her life), and it wasn't the best example. This is not to criticize my father or blame him, but rather to show what we as children learn from our parents, both healthy and unhealthy behaviors. I have to say I have met a handful of people who immediately knew right from wrong regarding their parents' unhealthy behaviors and made a choice to do better. I commend them, and even interviewed a few on my radio show in 2014. That wasn't my case. Decades passed and I experienced several life lessons before realizing right from wrong.

After I came home and we talked, we continued with couple's therapy. In our first session together after my affair, LL4 said that I had to do all the work because I had betrayed him. I said, "Yeah, I did, but this is both of us; we both have things we need to work on together." I felt like we were back to square one where I was putting in all the work versus both of us working through it together, and more importantly owning our reactions to any problems that arose between us. In February 2009, LL4 decided to leave home and stay at a hotel to get some time and space for himself. We had a date night, dinner out, and then we went back to his hotel room to hang out. He forced me to have sex often, and this was another time that he did. I was date raped by a guy I had a crush on when I was in high school, so I am a bit sensitive to being forced in the bedroom. Furthermore, we women need to be emotionally connected to our man to have pleasurable sex. I know I did not talk about this earlier. At age 16, I was forced to have sex for my very first time. It affected me well into my marriage. My therapist had to tell my husband that when your wife says no, it means no. At this point, our marriage was hanging by a thread. We had no emotional connection; no foundation.

We're great at falling in love but most aren't equipped to stay in love. Love is more than physical attraction and good sex. Marriage is working on getting to know one another and working every day on the relationship. It can often get dirty, it's not pretty, but that's real life.

In February, I was offered a job with VPX/Redline at the 2009 Arnold Sports Festival in Ohio. Airfare and hotel were paid for along with compensation for the three days I worked the fitness expo plus a per diem. This was a great opportunity seeing that VPX/Redline was a well-known reputable supplement company. LL4 would have attended this event with me except he had a work event that weekend. He was upset because he knew CA1 would be at the fitness event. So, at the expo, who do I see? CA1. It was March then and we talked for the first time since early January. We hung out at the after-party together, but went home to our separate hotels that night. And no, we did not have sex. The next day my flight home was canceled due to rain. I needed to be home for an appointment that Monday, so I ended up getting a ride home from CA1 and a friend whom I used to work with. They had driven to Ohio together for the expo. I still had strong feelings for CA1, especially since things with LL4 were pretty much the same. Later that same week, LL4 and I were having dinner alone at home, and I broke down crying. I told him I couldn't be a good wife, and that I had nothing left to give to him or our marriage. I came from a place of love, not anger or resentment. He responded by telling me he would stop drinking, that he refused to get a divorce, and that he would be a changed man.

He did stop drinking, but he had done this before numerous times in the nine years we were together. He stops and then weeks or months go by, and he starts up all over again. However, he was not arguing with me at all. He finally was not instigating or escalating situations. During this same time, CA1 and I started hanging out again in his area going to movies, visiting his family, and so on. Then one day we hung out around my area and people started seeing us together, which stressed me out, of course. I told him, "I can't do this anymore. If I leave my husband, I have to do it for the right reasons, and I can't have you as a crutch. If I have you there, it's too easy. I can't keep lying like this." So I cut CA1 off again, but he started begging to come back into my life. A week later I let him back in. Then a month went by, and he cut me off. He told me he wanted normalcy. He didn't want to have to hide "us." He wanted to live his life and follow his dreams by moving out west in hopes of building his modeling and acting career, and that now was not a good time for us. He said, "If we are going do this, we need to do it the right way; not like this. You do what you need to do, and I will do what I need to do, and if it is meant to be, we will be together again. If not, then we carry on in our lives."

In May, I again left home and spent time at a friend's. LL4 found a couple's retreat called Retrouvaille™ on www.retrouvaille.org. He said he wanted to attend and give us one last try. As for me, I am and always will be willing to give anything a try. I am open to learning and bettering myself. I went first and foremost to help me in my next relationship, and secondly for our marriage but I was done. As horrible as that may sound, I had hit my breaking point with LL4. We had a conversation before we went on the retreat. He said if we did work things out, he would like to renew our vows and have his mom give him away. That actually meant a lot that he was able to see the impact his mother had on our relationship and on him. His mother was a wonderful woman; however, when you marry you leave your parents for your spouse and that he did not do. He now understood that we as a couple came before his mother.

"When you marry, you form a new family unit. If you don't leave your parents, you can't fully cleave to your spouse." - @MarriageMentor on Twitter

I have had several friends, relatives, and clients ask for my professional advice regarding their marriages. I have highly encouraged each of them to seek help from a professional counselor and/or attend Retrouvaille™. It began in the seventies and is now in 150 counties, and the success rate is 85%, which is higher than marital counseling. The one weekend they had it in Chicago in May did not work with my schedule though. You are at the retreat location from Friday afternoon until Sunday. It is very intense, but worth it. We ended up flying to Tampa for the retreat. When we arrived, the body language of each couple from Friday to Sunday was completely different. Some couples were even staying in separate hotel rooms. It reminded me of how my parents lived under our roof growing up, in separate bedrooms most of the time. There were three couples that had been married 30+ years sharing their stories with us. The men told stories of 10-15 years ago, bawling about the affairs they had and how their wives forgave them, how they worked together, and moved forward in their marriages. One man even shared his story of alcoholism and how it negatively affected his marriage, that after years, he decided to attend AA, and how he and his wife worked hard to turn their marriage around from that point forward. Many couples in the room were crying. We did; LL4 and I could totally relate to each couple's story. Alcoholism and infidelity. They shared how they came to the retreat and held on a little longer for that miracle, and how they stayed together and fought hard for one another. They all waited for a miracle. The retreat also gave us more tools to fight fair in our marriage. Both nights we had homework. After a long day at the retreat, we went back to our room to work on the assignments given. Upon leaving they advised us that whatever decision we made regarding our marriage to be sure to sit down calmly and discuss it together...and be sure to hold on for a miracle.

When we finally returned home a few days later, LL4 said he wanted to go to AA. I was like, huh? Now? Really? For me, it was too late. I was in talks with a divorce lawyer and I was ready to move on in my life without him and without CA1. I received an invitation to be flown to Mexico City for a guest appearance in June and I accepted this once-in-a-lifetime offer. LL4 insisted on attending with me and being by my side the entire time. I was informed that I would have a body guard while I was there, so I wasn't concerned about my safety or having LL4 with me. Again, LL4 wanting to be a part of my life now was too late. It didn't matter. In the meantime, CA1 and I had become Facebook friends again. Yes, I just admitted that and included that in my book. LL4 saw this friendship and immediately confronted me at home. He was very upset, and rightfully so. There was nothing going on between us at that point though. We both just wanted to stay connected on "the book." LL4 and I got into a heated argument over it. At that point, I came clean and told him that I was meeting with my divorce attorney when I returned from Mexico City. I had planned to sit down with LL4 and have a calm adult conversation regarding my filing for divorce. I had never intended for it to come out in the middle of an argument, but it did. How many people actually have a calm discussion about getting a divorce?

Saving us

...it meant everything to me. I enabled him a lot. I didn't do anything. I did the same thing and got the same results. Consequences shape behavior. The thought of losing me changed LL4's behavior. I had been alone in our marriage for years and finally reached my breaking point. His reluctance to admit his problem destroyed our marriage. I had to do what I had to do for me. I couldn't be pulled down any longer. I know I hurt my husband; I, too, led to the demise of our relationship.

Our marriage was not horrible all the time. We had a lot of good times and shared great memories. I would not have married him if he were not a good person. He and I both turned outward in our marriage, instead of inward to each other. The tools given in both therapy and during the retreat help one to learn to speak or write their feelings. Adults are hurt children. We all enter relationships with wounds and if your partner can understand this, things will be easier. Whether the woman or the man tells you how they are feeling, it is about them and more often than not couples will cut one another off versus just listening from their hearts and hearing them out 100% on what is going on at that present moment and how they are feeling. So these tools teach you to be more compassionate and validate your partner's needs and feelings. I learned to make "I" statements versus "You" statements. For example, if upset or hurt, many will say "you do this" and "you do that", and "you-you-you." Essentially you are attacking the person. Whereas an "I" statement is telling your partner that, "I don't like when you do this or that," "it hurts my feelings," etc., or, "I love it when you do that," and "thank you, and I would appreciate if you did this or that more often." How many of you approach your partner in this manner? We are more likely to tear them down than to build them up. We typically say "You" versus "I." If we came from a loving place we would get more out of our relationships. That often requires being vulnerable, something we all need to practice and get more comfortable with. In other words, getting comfortable being uncomfortable. Therapy teaches you so much, if you are open to it. It taught me how to better listen to my partner and how to put myself in his shoes. It taught me how to better communicate my needs and emotions in a healthy manner, not just to men but to almost anyone in my life. Letter writing is a great tool to discuss problems and feelings. There is no yelling or screaming and you can reread what you wrote, erase any harsh words and revise it before giving it to your partner. When you speak without thinking, you can't take your words back. I highly recommend this tool. Most importantly, therapy helped me learn me.

About two weeks after I filed for divorce, LL4 started drinking again. He had brought another girl into our home with another couple and a guy friend. I woke up to find him passed out on the couch downstairs, lying next to her (they were fully clothed) with his hand on a glass of wine. At that point, I knew I had made the right decision. All along he had said he was changing for me. My response was, "Don't change for me, it won't last. You need to want to change for you and to be a better you." If he had truly wanted to change, he would have gone to AA regardless. I think he had brought her home to get a reaction out of me which it didn't. I knew what I had done to him, so how could I get mad? Why would I? I realized this was not about me and there was no need for me to react. So this would be a perfect example of being more present. Following this incident, he profusely apologized for bringing her into our house and said he would never do that again. The next month was so hard. He chased me around the house and tormented me. One minute he was trying to hug and kiss me, the next he was saying the meanest, cruelest things to me. I often locked myself in our master bathroom to get away from him. Needless to say, he moved downtown in August of 2009, which was a blessing. It was too hard for both of us to be around one another. Rejection isn't easy; I was rejecting him, so I do not blame him for his behavior. I understood it-- not that I would say it was healthy and acceptable, but I was able to put myself in his shoes. There was no reason for me to react to him by being mean back or being vindictive. I had hurt him enough.

"I hit a cross. I was bearing a cross. I was in conflict with my sin. Identify with Jesus Christ. Deal with sin. It may not be something you want to do. Like how Jesus didn't want to go to the cross. Translation: I don't want to deal with this. This thing hurts, it's difficult. You have to make a conscious decision to pick up your cross. Skip me! I don't want to deal. Your feelings, your pain, your situation is real. Feelings don't think that's why they change. All you need is new information for your feelings to change. Face your sin." - Tony Evans

If you have been married to an addict, had or have a parent or sibling who was or is an alcoholic or had other addictions, then you can easily relate. I have had many conversations with people on this topic. Some have not been involved with someone with an addiction so they cannot relate. When you have an addiction, that is your priority. No person, place or thing comes before it. Addicts surround themselves with others who use or they often use alone.

"Wounds don't heal until they're witnessed. If you're stuck in denial, your secrets will remain locked in your cells, unavailable for witnessing and healing." - Dr. Christiane Northrup, M.D.

Glory Jordan, Our Marital Counselor, 2005 - 2009

When working with people, they must understand that they can't change a person; they need to understand that they need to work on themselves. I feel people should take couples therapy and it should be a class in schools, too. Go to <u>www.selfleadership.org</u>; there is a great model on my site to help you make changes that last. I trained in this model, too.

We try to get into the relationship to help them make the changes they need to create a better relationship. We try to get people to turn into their own self power to make these changes within their own life. People at times have a hard time understanding that they can't change a person to be who they want them to be. The person has to want to change to be a better person. Therapy helps people to look at both sides as to one side of the relationship. I always say relationships are for a season and a reason.

A lot of people come into a relationship with wounded parts, and once we learn from these parts we can address them. Every relationship will have these parts and if we don't learn from this, we will repeat the same relationship. It's like wherever you leave off on with your last relationship, you tend to pick up with the next relationship, unless you address them. Every person has issues they need to work on, so if a person doesn't stop and address their own self issues they will bring them into the next relationship, creating another unhealthy relationship. It is a shame that there is not insurance for couple's counseling because it is really needed.

There is a lot of good information in the book on that website. If they had relationship counseling taught in the high schools, it would help a lot. I don't know anyone that had a great childhood. They may "think" they did, but that is where it starts. We need to build self-worth in children, and work on family issues to create better self-esteem.

At times I have learned that working with people as a couple works great when you keep them apart. If they are in the room together they will react to each other's answers. It is always great to keep the couple together since it is a relationship but both ways are beneficial.

A few things Glory taught us on healthy fighting:
1- Remain in the present.
2- Eliminate blame, name calling, put downs and hostile judgements.
3- Avoid score-keeping.
4- Focus on solving the problem.

5- *Accept ownership of your part of the problem.*
6- *Manage your feelings, especially your anger.*
7- *Practice empathy...how your partner feels.*
8- *Don't assume, ask.*
9- *Avoid aggressive, passive or passive aggressive communications.*
10- *Seek to understand the other person first, then to be understood.*

Marriage is not part time, it's not full time; it's all the time, 110% of the time, even when you don't want it to be. If people put that same time and energy into their relationships as they did their careers, the divorce rate would drop. People just don't have the tools. There is no school on emotions, there is no school on parenting, and there is no school on relationships. There are workshops and seminars, but that is it.

Divorce is so common. What is the definition of marriage when your mother and father divorce? When a brother divorces? Hmmm. Infidelity is quite common too. My mom caught my father having an affair. I have a half aunt and half uncle because my grandfather had an affair with his secretary. My grandmother knew too. He was raising two families at the same time. However, I did not find this out until 2005, many years after both my grandparents had passed. All along, I thought my grandparents had the perfect relationship, the perfect marriage. Ha, was I wrong! There is no such thing. Couples need to work hard at their relationships each and every year. Marriage is a work-in-progress. I quit my marriage, and I turned outward to another man. I did not have the tools. Now I do. This doesn't mean my life and relationships going forward will be perfect. It just means I know better how to set boundaries, what I need to overcome and not run from, and when to ask for help if I need it.

"Men choose their wives for the way they are, they don't want anything to change, and do not realize that women often want change. Women choose their husbands for characteristics they possess, and most importantly because of the potential they see in their mate. They hope to change them to make them the man they think they can be. This helps to achieve a greater than 50% divorce rate in America and the fact that many women will change, frustrating their husbands, and many men won't, frustrating their wives."- Unknown

Focusing On Me

"Failure is success if we learn from it." - Paul V Harris

My marriage and divorce were a success; I learned so much!

When you are going through a hard time in life, it is so easy to shut down and push people away. I did push people away because I knew they were toxic, I did not want to be around them, or I just wanted to be alone. It's amazing what you can accomplish when you eliminate draining, negative, incompatible, not-going-anywhere relationships or friendships. My mother, brother, and a few others knew that I had filed for divorce. I had kept this on the D.L. (down low). Even though this was something I had wanted, it was still excruciatingly painful; more painful than my father's death. A divorce is essentially a death. From then on, I focused on myself and my career, and for once in my life, I didn't date someone right away. When life knocks you down, it either fuels you to shut down or to crank it up a notch and power through.

Love yourself enough to date yourself before adding another. Never force anything, especially when it isn't working.

My career started to take off. A funny story: before I left for Miami to compete in June 2009, I was with a girlfriend at a local bar. I was not drinking since I was competing that following weekend. A member of the gym where I work was trying very hard to persuade me to have shots with him. I did not know him; he just knew me from the gym since I worked there. Of course, he was wasted. I looked at him and asked, "If you had a goal and I tried to sabotage it, what would you do?" He shut up. After capturing the title of the 2009 Ms. Bikini Classic Universe, this guy apologized when I returned to work after hearing my news. He even complimented me later on my career and how he had seen a lot of my work online. Stay strong people! Never let anyone sabotage your goals or bully you!

I then decided to compete in a different federation, the NPC/ IFBB Bikini Division, that fall. The International Federation of Bodybuilding and Fitness is the most prestigious federation in the world and I was scared I would fail. I not only captured a world title, but I was promoting Chicago shows for Fitness/ Bikini Universe. I had to give that up, promoting a show for a different federation, so I could compete with another. Only makes sense right? That also meant losing out on a lot of money each year that we made promoting the Chicago show. I entered my first NPC (National Physique Committee) bikini competition in September and won. The NPC is the amateur division of the IFBB. Following that, I went to my first national show placing sixth. I was also flown out again to California for TV commercial jobs and still under contract for more modeling with VPX/Redline. All of this gave me a lot of exposure, which helped my personal training business too. It wasn't until the fall/ winter of 2009 that I finally started to open up to others and share my divorce. Another reason I didn't share it with many is because I just didn't want any men asking me out. I needed to be alone to grieve and work on myself.

"Being single gives you the opportunity to practice self-reliance." - Gentlemenhood on Twitter

When LL4 and I got married, I wanted to give both my mom and mother-in-law (at the time) tickets to *Oprah* at our rehearsal dinner. My mom loved her and watched every show. She tape recorded the shows she missed. In 2005, I was not able to get the both of them any tickets. However, in 2009, a client had told me they emailed in and got tickets right away. So I tried again and this time, I did get two tickets to her show on Michigan Avenue. However, it was standing room only, and the *Oprah Show* had a stated plan to be there 4-6 hours. Well, my mom had knee-replacement surgery and couldn't walk or stand for long periods of time. So being the vocal person I am, I emailed them and asked if they had any special accommodations for those with special needs, like my mom with her knee. They then told me where to go upon arrival. When we arrived, I valet parked, and then we were greeted and escorted into this amazing event. They had blocked off several streets for it. I remember several others who were going but were lost in the crowd (yes, I am rubbing it in). I pushed my mom in her wheelchair most of the way and we finally landed in our seats: front row! Yes, front row, left of the stage; they had an area blocked off for those with requests like ours. Needless to say, I was glad I was able to give my mom the gift of Oprah, front row and all. We had a great time and she took a lot of pictures as usual. For the first time in my life, I was happy that my mom struggled with getting around and had knee problems. If not, we would not have had the experience we did.

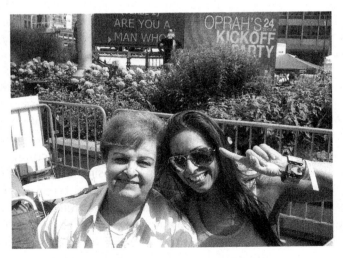

Mary & Nicole Moneer at Oprah

The economy tanked when we were trying to sell our house in 2009. Our $500,000 home had dropped in value $150,000. In 2010, we decided it was best to foreclose since we had not received an offer in a year's time. Since LL4 moved out in August of 2009, he gave up his rights to live in our home. My mom brought one of her male friends over on Thanksgiving, and he was giving me such a hard time regarding our foreclosure. He knew nothing about my marriage or my situation, yet he was so upset we were foreclosing on our home. This was my first time meeting him too! He kept asking me all these questions, telling me what I should and shouldn't do. I never asked for his advice. Don't you love those "types" of people? He put a bad taste in my mouth, and I never wanted to be around him again. I did not stress about our foreclosure. I could have listed a dozen other things that could have happened to me that would have been a lot worse. If this was the worst thing that was going to happen to me right now, I'd take it, and I would recover. I did not have to worry about rent; I lived there rent free for two years. After receiving the final foreclosure notice, I did move out, and was able to rent. My credit was excellent before our foreclosure and after, it really wasn't as bad as I would have thought since I beat others out on the rental property. In the end, it all worked out in my favor.

I needed my husband LL4, and I am forever grateful for the years of marriage counseling we had. Glory was the best therapist in my opinion, plus I was ready to change. LL4 was a gift in my life. With that being said, I don't want him back in my life. I know how much I hurt him and I am truly sorry. After my divorce, I had many people reaching out to me for advice regarding their marriages with the same story as ours. Many admitted to me that they were having affairs. I told LL4 that when he came to our house in 2011 to pick up some of his belongings he had left. I told him that I wanted to open a school for marriage and parenting. LL4 replied, "Nicole you can't teach anyone what we learned." So true and profound.

Then came LL5

"There is nothing more beautiful than a person whose heart has broken but who still believes in love." - Unknown

As soon as I told my best guy friend about my big "D," LL5 texted me. LL5 was best friends with my guy friend, hence him finding out the news of my divorce. We ended up dating for a few months and had a lot of fun together. He was at a place in his life where he was not ready for a relationship based on all he had been through and what he was currently going through at the time we dated. He thought he was at first, but don't a lot of people? The reason I even mention LL5 is because I came out a winner after our time together. For the first time in my dating career, I was better able to put myself in his shoes. I could better communicate my feelings in a healthy manner, and I started to ask the right questions. Once he communicated to me (which didn't happen for months), I understood where he had been and all he had been through, and that he needed to work through his issues on his own. Knowing where I have been and all I have been through, I am proud of how I handled myself during the time we dated and after. I was in a much better place. We are still friends today; he is a good soul.

During the time we dated, I competed in Bikini in the Arnold Amateur in 2010 and I placed second. Every year, bodybuilders, physique, figure and bikini competitors compete in the amateur and pro shows that are part of The Arnold Fitness Festival. I was flabbergasted at how high I placed in this contest. People started to recognize me from my VPX/Redline ad that was published in every national fitness magazine. In May, bodybuilding.com hired me to work the UFC Fan Expo in Las Vegas and in June of 2010, my divorce finalized. I then competed in my second National Physique Committee national show and placed fifth. Believe it or not, I was not happy with this placing. I wanted and expected to win. Doesn't everyone? I was considering not competing in another two weeks at Team Universe because I was so upset about my placing. I had spoken to the head judge and received her invaluable feedback. She told me I needed to work on my butt and change my suit color. I was so insulted! My butt was my best body part. I was really ticked off. Needless to say, I sucked it up, worked my booty off, and decided to compete in Team U in New Jersey. Well, I am so glad I did. I was awarded my pro card in the IFBB Bikini Division. I share this and many other stories with my female clients who compete. I tell them to never expect a win, to stay positive of course, to set goals, and to keep their heads out of their asses. I tell them to never quit; if you give something a try or one more try, you never know where it might lead you. I also tell many to grow a thick skin and learn lots of patience, no matter what their life journey. Judges' feedback and having a second eye is so important; we all have room for improvement.

For those of you not familiar with The International Federation of Body Builders, becoming a part of this elite iconic group is quite an accomplishment. It is quite an honor to become a professional. At this time, I was not dating anyone and happy with me, myself, and I. I was still personal training at LifeTime Fitness and traveling to compete and work for both VPX/Redline and bodybuilding.com on weekends here and there. VPX hired me to work their booth at the 2009 Olympia which is held in Las Vegas yearly. The following year, bodybuilding.com hired me to work their booth at the 2010 Olympia. I was later hired on to be a part of the 2011 bodybuilding.com inaugural team, which traveled to shows all over the world promoting health and fitness. 2011 was a great year. I represented bodybuilding.com in Germany at the international fitness and wellness expo FIBO, I worked for VPX/Redline two weeks during the Indy 500, supported our military for both of these companies in 2010 and 2011, and received my Bikini Olympia qualification in November of 2011. The Olympia is the Olympics of bodybuilding. The best of the best in the world compete; men's and women's bodybuilding, women's fitness, figure and bikini. They recently added a women's and men's physique division as well.

Another highlight of my career to add to my resume: my personal training business was really taking off as well. I want to take a moment and give thanks for all the opportunities given to me and where they have led me today. On my flight to Germany, bodybuilding.com teammate, Nick Scott, and I discussed my interest in writing a book. As an author, he was a wealth of knowledge. I asked him a few questions so I too could accomplish a dream of writing my own book. He told me to just start writing, so when I got home, I did. I got one page done and then another, and then another. In December of 2011, I received an email from a publishing company. An anonymous fan of mine had given them some of my story and told them to contact me. I wasn't sure if this email was legit so I forwarded it to Nick and he sent me back some questions to ask them. After looking at my emails, Nick confirmed this was a legit deal and to hop on it.

I often tell people be careful what you post on social media. You never know who is watching and/or what amazing opportunities may come your way.

We went back and forth regarding my publishing contract until March 2012. I remember the day well. The day I finalized the book contract was the same day my mother died, unexpectedly.

Chapter 5 - Losing My Mom

"My mother was the most beautiful woman I ever saw. All I am, I owe to my mother. I attribute all my success in life to the moral, intellectual, and physical education I received from her." - George Washington.

I also contribute my success, independence, and high self-esteem in life to the unconditional love my mother gave me. She gave me her time, her acceptance, and her constant loving presence. You cannot put a price on that. It's what all children need from both parents.

My aunt, Barbara (remember, the one I visited in NYC while in high school), had called and said that my mom had died. She, along with my other aunt, found her at her house. After I received the call, I was obviously in a state of shock, numb but at the same time, I knew what to expect having lost my father 16 years prior. Since my brother lived in California, I knew I would be responsible again for her estate, which seemed overwhelming. At 39, I was emotionally in a better place regarding the other "D" word, death. That did not mean her death came easy; I just had a better understanding of death and how to handle the situation as far as what all needed to be taken care of that first week and the months and year following. My aunts found her on Sunday, March 11. I had last spoken to her on Saturday, March 10. Somehow God told me to call her, and I am so glad I did. I was heading to a massage appointment at my chiropractor of 10 years at the time. I was actually returning my mom's call from two days prior. We spoke briefly. When she answered the phone, she sounded like hot piss. It was 1 pm when I called but you would have thought it was 1 am and I had woken her from a deep sleep the way she sounded. I asked what was wrong. She said that she had worked the last couple of days and was tired. I thought nothing of it. My mother never told me anything regarding her health. When I arrived at her home, my two aunts were there, along with my uncle and two of my mom's best friends. It was horrible. There she was, in her recliner, dead. My brother and uncle were calling since they lived out of state. The funeral home staff arrived at her home that same day, and we immediately had to pick out an outfit for her jewelry and undergarments. I was so overwhelmed. This did not happen when my father died. My aunt, Beverly, my mom's best friend of 50 years with whom she went to nursing school, helped me. This was not an easy task considering the amount of clothes and jewelry my mother had. It was so hard to pick one outfit and a few pieces of jewelry that she would be buried in. The wake was scheduled for Friday that week which gave my brother and uncle enough time to travel in.

I remember that week well. Sunday night I did not sleep a wink. I texted LL4 that day to inform him about my mother's death. He was really upset. We were up in the middle of the night texting one another. That Monday I asked my aunt, Barbara, to come with me to the funeral home to make arrangements. This time it was definitely a different experience with my mother not being Muslim, a positive one, but so much to select and choose from. My brother and I requested an autopsy be done; we wanted answers. Based on the pathologist report, she died on Saturday, which I knew in my gut happened after our phone call. She had an enlarged heart and suffered a myocardial infarction. She had heart problems, like my father did. The heart is all about our emotions and neither of my parents excelled at handling their emotions. Having lost both my parents to the number one killer in America, I researched more on it and found this:

From heartmath.org

"75 to 90% of all visits to primary care physicians result from stress-related disorders." - Paul Rosch, M.D., President, American Institute of Stress

Another study in this section assesses changes in the levels of two essential hormones, DHEA and cortisol, in a group of people who practiced a Heart-Math emotional management intervention over one month's time. DHEA, known as the "anti-aging hormone," is the precursor to the human sex hormones estrogen and testosterone. Its varied physiological effects include enhancing the immune system, stimulating bone deposition, lowering cholesterol levels and building muscle mass. DHEA has been found to be deficient in individuals who suffer from many diseases, including obesity, diabetes, hypertension, cancer, Alzheimer's, immune deficiency, coronary artery disease and various autoimmune disorders. Cortisol, a glucocorticoid hormone, is involved in protein, carbohydrate and fat metabolism and is widely known as the "stress hormone" because it is secreted in excessive amounts when people are under stress.

Separate studies showed that the risk of developing heart disease is significantly increased for people who impulsively vent their anger as well as for those who tend to repress angry feelings. - A. Siegman et al. J Behav M.Ed. 1998; 21(4) D. Carroll et al. J Epidemiol Comm Health. 1998; Sept.

In a groundbreaking study of 1,200 people at high risk of poor health, those who learned to alter unhealthy mental and emotional attitudes through self-regulation training were more than 4 times more likely to be alive 13 years later than an equal-sized control group. - R. Grossarth-Maticek and H. Eysenck. Behav Res Ther. 1991; 29(1)

"We are coming to understand health not as the absence of disease, but rather as the process by which individuals maintain their sense of coher-

ence (i.e. sense that life is comprehensible, manageable and meaningful) and ability to function in the face of changes in themselves and their relationships with their environment." - Aaron Antonovsky (1987). Unraveling the Mystery of Health: How People Manage Stress and Stay Well.

In recent years a number of investigators have proposed the DHEA/cortisol ratio to be an important biological marker of stress and aging. When individuals are under prolonged stress, a divergence in this ratio results, as cortisol levels continue to rise while DHEA levels decrease significantly. The effects of DHEA/cortisol imbalance can be severe, and may include elevated blood sugar levels, increased bone loss, compromised immune function, decreased skin repair and regeneration, increased fat accumulation and brain cell destruction.

The Physiological and Psychological Effects of Compassion and Anger

Key findings: Heart-focused, sincere, positive feeling states boost the immune system, while negative emotions may suppress the immune response for up to six hours following the emotional experience.

I love this from Dr. Christiane Northrup:

Adopt the attitude that everything that happens to you- especially if you've been wronged- has a reason that you sometimes can't see. Be willing to go along with it and be as gracious as possible. Sometimes you have to accept the unacceptable. When you do so, your cells won't suffer and neither will your immune system- and you'll feel a lot better.

Emotions take a huge toll on the body. I have experienced it myself many times in my 40 years. I see it in my clients and even in my brother's health. Most of the time, I am teaching clients how to rest more. I prescribe adrenal tests, and yoga and Pilates days. I even encourage them to clean up the negative toxic, draining people in their lives. So many things affect the health of our hearts. In August 2008, when my ex-husband left home for about two weeks, I was destroyed emotionally. At that time, I went in to my integrative doctor to get a MSA test. My liver and small intestines were always stressed, showing up in the red. This time my heart was in the red. My doctor knew nothing about my situation at home. This test proves how much stress can negatively affect your organs, your heart health and overall health. He did give me homeopathic remedies which did strengthen my heart, along with my own emotional healing that took place following.

My mom was on various medications, none of which I was made aware of until her death. Neither of my parents ever shared their health with my brother or me. Ironically, I could have helped my mother turn her health around had she wanted my help. However, I was at peace because she never asked for my help. Some people don't want it. They are perfectly content living their lives as is, even if they are in pain. I knew there was nothing that I could have done to change her health. Only she could make that change, no one else. God wanted her, her time here on earth was done and now she was at peace. That Monday night, I was exhausted. I finally slept that night. My cousin, Julie, and my boss at LifeTime Fitness, DJ, had both called me on Monday. My boss asked if I would attend our weekly team meeting so that the team could embrace me during such a difficult time and give me hugs. I about lost it. How many of you have a boss who would even think to ask you this? He called me every day that week to make sure I was alright. How many of you have a boss who would check up on you daily? When my father died, I isolated myself, which is very normal after losing a loved one. This time I opened up and allow myself to be vulnerable. I accepted his gracious invitation and attended our meeting briefly. I felt good after that meeting. I did not think I would have the strength to go to my work two days after my mom died, but I did. Here is an interview my publisher had with my former boss, DJ:

DJ (LifeTime Fitness Personal Training Department Head, 2012)

I was Nicole's boss over a year ago, and I was promoted over to the club as a department head; this was how we met. Nicole already had a full client schedule, and was very professional. She knew what she wanted and didn't want; she was very seasoned. She is a very hard worker, and can juggle a lot of different things in the professional world and in her personal life.

One thing about Nicole is her laugh. Once you hear it, you will never forget it. She was always business, but she had a way to put smiles on peoples' faces. She dealt with the passing of her mom extremely well, better than most people. As a team we did try to give her that support. She needed to work and to keep her mind focused; she never brought the passing of her mom to work, and that was what stuck out the most.

One of the things I would like the reader to know about Nicole is how down to earth she really is. People see the pretty face and all the things she has accomplished and would think she is cocky or stuck up, but she is far from it. She is a real people person and she cares about people as a whole. Overall, Nicole is a very passionate person about health and fitness, and is very intelligent.

I was very touched by what DJ had to say about me, and how he reached out to me that week. We still keep in touch to this day. He has been promoted several times within LifeTime Fitness. I am sure you can see just one reason why. Back to my mom's death: that week my cousin asked if I wanted to spend the day with her three daughters. Children; another dose of good medicine. I again accepted this offer. When I arrived at their house later that afternoon, the three girls were outside playing basketball. It was 80 degrees on this day in March, a rare occurrence in Chicago. The youngest, Ava, ran up to the car to give me a hug. She was four years old at the time. I cried and embraced her for a long time. To this day, every time we see each other at family events, she runs up to me and hugs me. Later on the girls asked if we could go play at the park, so off we went in mom's mini-van. They were in the back and mom and I in the front. Out of nowhere they start calling me "Picky Nicky." My cousin and I look at each other, and I turned around and looked at them like, "Huh?" They had never ever called me this, ever. My mom called me Nicky Picky and Picky Nicky ever since I was a little girl. My mom was in the car that day. When we got to the park, we played on the swings and enjoyed being outdoors. It was such a treat.

Tuesday night I did not sleep. On Wednesday, I spoke with my marital counselor for a good hour. One thing she said that I remember was that I should not be surprised if my mom comes to talk to me. It happens often when a loved one dies. She said she may come through a book or some other way. Wednesday night, my Brother Anonymous arrived home after midnight. I was too exhausted to pick him up. I was at a point where I just couldn't do it all anymore. I called my uncle, Jerry; he has been a rock for our family so many times. He was my rock that night. I broke down crying, saying I needed my sleep and that I could not pick my brother up. I asked if he could, so he did. On Thursday, I drove to my mother's home and met with my uncle, John, my mom's brother who had arrived in town. I selected photos for viewing at her wake. I needed to leave in the afternoon to head back to pick up my brother for our appointment with the priest to review details for the funeral. When I got in my car, I checked my cell phone (before driving) and read an email from my cousin, Julie. When I opened it, this was the picture she sent me of her daughter Ava, with this book:

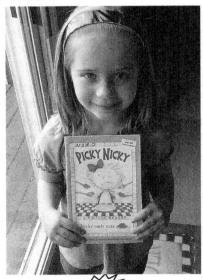

After I saw this picture, I literally laughed and laughed and laughed. This was my mom talking to me; she wanted me to be happy, not sad. My mom had a great sense of humor and loved to laugh. Every time I see Ava to this day, I feel the presence of my mother in her. She hugs me so tight, I love it. My mom did the same too. Ava is my little angel.

When talking with the priest on Thursday, we went over songs for the mass. We also talked about my mom. My brother had memories of when he was in the bubble in Seattle and how mom was with him every day, playing chess. My brother broke down crying telling the story to the priest, as did I listening to him. Our mother was always there for us no matter what. Such fond memories. Then the big day came; Friday, my mom's wake. My best friend, Jennifer, the same one who took me in at her house when I needed a place to stay back in January 2009 after the shit hit the fan regarding my marriage, had flown in from Las Vegas to be there for me. I did not even ask her. She saw my post on Facebook and called me. Thank God for Facebook in this matter because that is how most of our family and friends found out. Jen was my rock during this time; she was a rock for us all. She stayed at my place along with my brother, his fiancée and his fiancée's daughter, and I am so grateful for her and all she has done for me. She is such a selfless person. She drove us Friday and Saturday. Those of you who have lost a loved one know wakes and funerals are difficult enough; there is no way my brother or I could have driven either of those days. At the wake, my mom's pastor spoke. I wanted to and did, as did my brother and our uncle (my mom's brother). Surprisingly, I had the strength to speak. At my dad's wake, I was a mess and there was no way I could let out a peep. It was funny; her pastor shared with us how he would receive Christmas cards in the summer from my mom with pictures of her daughter in bikinis. My mom loved me and was very proud of me. I had a good relationship with her and I knew she loved me. We both told each other this, and I know all of this made her death easier for me to cope with. That week flew by, and then my brother, Jennifer, and my uncle flew back home.

I played "Say" by John Mayer, over and over the week of her death. I still do when I'm driving in my car. It makes me bawl. Crying is good; grieving is good. There is no timeline on grief. It also made me realize I did "say" all I needed to, to my mom. We both did. I didn't need closure to tell her I loved and appreciated her and all she did for me; she already knew, and vice versa. She always showed me and told me how much she loved me and how proud of me she was.

It was very difficult for me to go to her bank. I didn't for at least two months following her death. I cried in my car in the parking lot; I couldn't even go in. I started walking in and was bawling. I had to turn around and sit in my car to calm down a bit. Some people would be happy thinking, "Oh yippee, money," but I was hurting. I always phone first so I have all the needed information beforehand to make sure I don't have any problems. When I called her bank, they told me I needed this and that, which I brought. Not true; they had given me the run around. Banks need to better educate their staff as to how to deal with death. They sent me home three times to get more of this and that. It was hard enough dealing with my mom's death, and now I had to deal with the bank. A friend suggested I go to another branch, so I did and I had no problems. They took care of me that day, no questions asked.

Every weekend for a year I went to her house and cleaned it. Never once did I go alone; that is how many angels I have in my life. Thank you again to all of you; you know who you are. Saaema, my best friend since diapers and her younger sister, Heena, came that first weekend following her funeral. They were my good luck charms, my rocks when my dad died, and again my rocks when my mom died.

With their help we found her will and her car keys. It took us two weeks to find these very important things. Yes, that is how much crap my mom had in her house; a house filled with 69 years of crap.

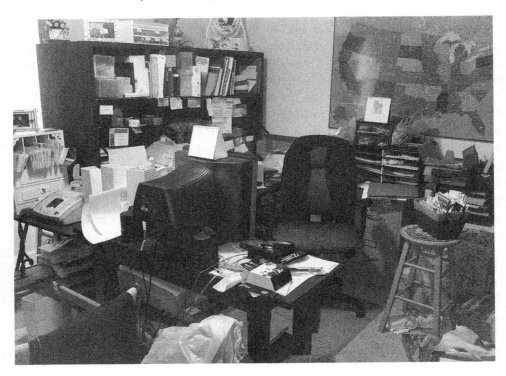

We all called my mom a pack rat; she even called herself this! The sad part was the food; the cookies and chocolate. She had food hidden everywhere throughout the house. From what I could tell she was depressed and turned to food as an outlet. I had no clue. It was sad to discover this.

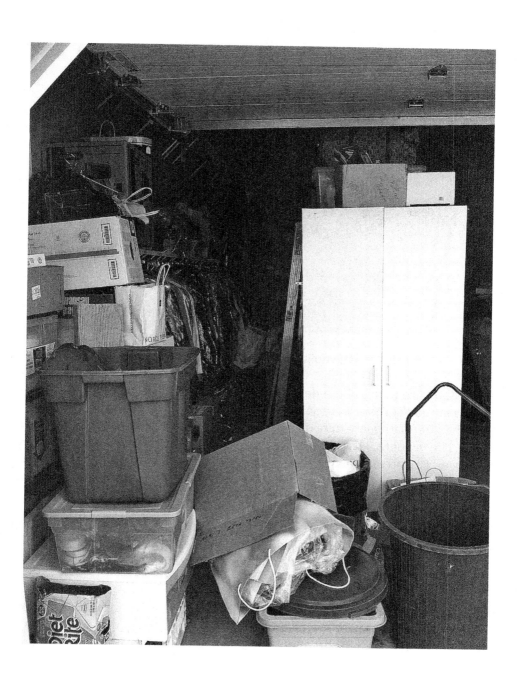

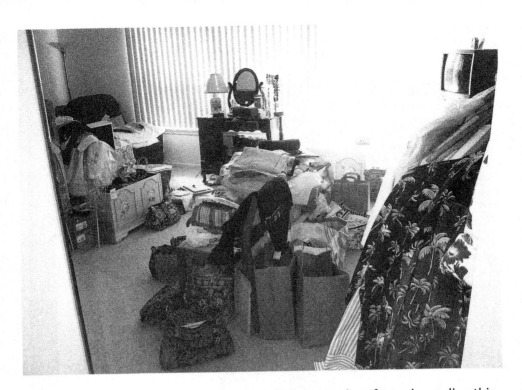

No one plans for the worst; you just don't. There are a lot of people reading this that will leave someone behind. Get your will together, and talk about it. I know people don't like to talk about death, but my mom's will was never updated, the same as my dad's. There were some issues with the will and the trust and this made the aftermath more difficult for us, especially me. People need to plan their estates. Life happens. I know we can't plan for everything, but death is something we all need to plan for. So make note, whoever your loved ones are, be sure you ask where they keep their will. Most people do not like to discuss death. However, it definitely makes it easier for those left behind.

I had to dig deep every week and get in my car to drive 45 minutes to her house to clean it. Once I was there though, I actually found a lot of peace and comfort in going through her belongings. We had a lot of fun, and we found a ton of money each week which actually paid for her garbage; yes, her garbage!

In her town, residents are required to buy stickers for each box or bag of garbage. Literally, my mom was haunting us. She never wanted to throw things out while alive and now deceased, it cost about $90-100 a week in stickers. That is how much garbage that would be piled curbside.

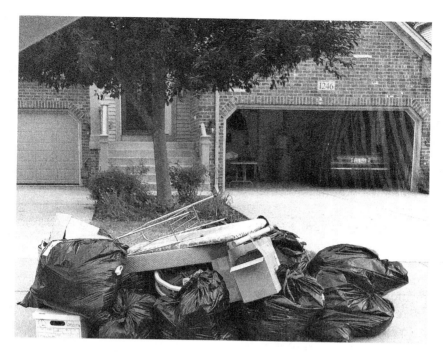

Thank goodness for all the cash we found stashed in all sorts of places in her home. I even took pictures in case people didn't believe me. The first time I went to Goodwill later that summer and dropped off a ton of my mom's belongings, I broke down crying.

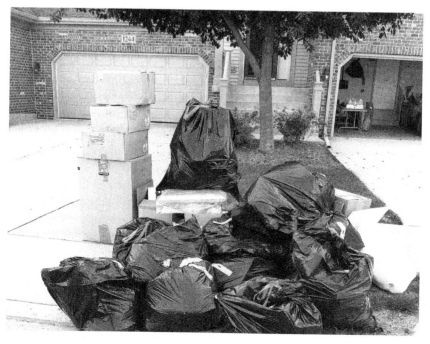

Easter 2012, I pulled my uncle, Jerry, aside, and cried thanking him for all he had done for my mom and our family over the years. My relatives rock!

In May, I decided to compete in Pittsburgh. I wasn't competing to win or place; I was competing as a much needed get-away from all of this and to hang with some of my fit friends from around the globe. Then in mid-June, I hosted athlete interviews for *Muscle and Fitness Hers* at a yearly bodybuilding, fitness, figure, bikini, and physique competition here in Chicago. On the last night of the event, I ran into CA1. Remember him from back in 2009? On and off over the past few years he would text me here and there, but nothing more. We hugged and caught up, and then said goodbye. Later that week I get a text from him, and we start talking again. We picked up right where we had left off. He asked me for another chance; he told me he was ready for a relationship and to move back home to Chicago. He wanted to come visit me, so he flew in just after the 4th of July and stayed six days. I had breast augmentation scheduled the day he was flying back to NYC. While he was here, we spent a few days with his family and worked out. He even helped clean my mom's home. We went to Navy Pier and had a really great time together. He decided at the last minute to stay another week and take care of me after my surgery. Okay, he had me hook, line and sinker when he decided to stay and take care of me. My mom's best friend of 50 years, Beverly, was going to help take care of me along with a client who had become a very close friend at the time. Instead, he took care of me. He met both of them the day of my surgery but the days following they still came. We talked about marriage. Actually he brought it up, and even told my friend and my mom's best friend he planned to marry me and throw a 40th birthday party for me in November. CA1 was going above and beyond for me; it wasn't just words, it was actions. He introduced me to this social media site called Instagram. I really had no clue how to use it and interact with others at the time, besides posting pictures on my profile.

After CA1 returned home, I was to visit him next out east in August. Instead, he surprised me with a visit two weeks later saying he missed me a ton. We had a good time again, but we had an argument or two, and I remember specifically that he and his mother had gotten into it. He told her to "F" off at the top of his lungs at my house while he was on the phone with her. CA1 proclaims to be "godly" on all of his social media posts. I am sorry, but godly people do not talk to their mother the way he did. She was upset because he posted a picture of his four year old nephew who was in the hospital with cancer. His picture had gotten 9,000 likes which was exactly what he wanted: the likes. His mom was upset that he posted something private regarding their family just for "fame" and popularity. He did not talk to his mom for a good two weeks because of this. I also would turn on Moody radio while in the car with him and he would say, "No way are we going to listen to this." Moody is a leading source of Christian talk radio. So again, CA1 pretends to be someone he is not on social media. If he is all about God, especially posting it to thousands of people, why would he be against listening to biblical talk? It makes me want to puke that hundreds of thousands believe him and actually look up to him. I started to see more evil in him; more of his devilish side. He would shoot up in front of me all the time, steroids that is. I am a 100% natural fitness and bikini competitor and always have been. He also sells steroids but keeps that under-cover. I know a few guys who he screwed over.

He returned home back east after a few days with me. I then traveled out to visit him in mid-August. After that, the plan was for him to come back to Chicago and stay for a good month, help me train for the 2012 Bikini Olympia and fly with me to another IFBB competition two weeks prior to the Olympia. He always mentioned moving back permanently to live with me since he was in sales with this supple-ment company and could work from anywhere. So I was with him for a long week-end in mid-August and we worked a fitness competition together. He was working for a new supplement company and they had a booth at this event. We were talk-ing with a lot of people at the event and taking a lot of pictures as well. Because of our following, we both decided to keep our relationship on the down low, he obvi-ously for other reasons than I; he is a player, especially with brunette bikini com-petitors and fitness models. I prefer to keep my relationships off social media for a plethora of reasons. Privacy is hard to come by in today's world. While we were there, I had his phone in my hand. I saw a text from a girl with a Las Vegas area code that said, "You were missed last night." I gave him his phone and asked who she was. He said thanks for asking and not assuming; she was a friend. Well I kept her name in my head. I headed back to Chicago and the plan was for him to fly back about five days later. He came up with all these excuses why he couldn't fly back to Chicago to be with me, like he had to work or had a photo shoot and so on. At first, I understood, but then I thought, "Something smells fishy", because he never did end up flying back. I started to creep his Instagram page and then this other girl's page. Yes, yes, I admit it; I too am a creeper, but not the creepy kind. I was just creeping for information. It was such intense research! Turns out they had been talking ever since he and I reconnected in July; no, not just talking like friends but posting comments under each other's pictures that were sexual or implying much more than a friendship. However, when I started on Instagram, I had no idea how to use it. Anyway, I didn't do anything. I played along with his game. He con-tinued to purposely be horribly mean to me and blow me off, hoping I would end things which would be the easy way out for him. I didn't. Then he started to turn things on me, blaming me for everything. Typical manipulator. He was even having episodes on the phone with me where he would be driving around raging because he couldn't find needles to shoot up; a side of him I had never seen. It was like he was addicted... a-dick-ted. What I did next was, well, immature, but I couldn't re-sist.

"Don't mistake my kindness for weakness. I am kind to everyone, but when someone is unkind to me, weak is not what you are going to remember about me." - Al Capone

The same day I flew to St. Louis for my last IFBB Pro Show before The Olympia, he posted a picture of himself at the airport heading west. Of course this other girl posted hearts under his picture. That night I got a text from him apologizing, stating he was ready to talk to me and that it wasn't fair of him to leave me hanging without any explanation. He wished me luck in my competition and said if I didn't want to talk that night, he understood. Later he posted a picture with himself, her and another guy friend at the pool where she worked, stating how beautiful she was and that she was taken. He did the same with me. I decided to contact her on her Model Mayhem account, a portfolio website for professional models. You could not send someone a private message on Instagram at the time and she did not have a private message option on Facebook. I told her I was looking for booth models in Las Vegas for an upcoming event and that I would be in town in two weeks to interview her if interested. There was some truth to this as I have referred several friends in the industry for well-paid, legitimate modeling jobs. However, in sending this message, I was messing with her, only to mess with him. I had no ill will towards her; he was the jerk. Soon after I hit the "Send" button, CA1 blocked me on Facebook. Ahhhh, the block button! I am actually going to change his name to Slimeball #1 (SB1) right now.

He always spoke ill of past girlfriends. Don't most guys, especially players? They are always trying to put themselves in a good light in front of other women. I know she told him I sent the message and asked if he knew me so I am sure he told her I was a crazy ex-girlfriend. Here I was, in such a vulnerable place having lost my mother, and he came back into my life, taking advantage of me. Sure I always wondered "what if" we had another chance, so I am glad we had that chance for many reasons, if only to prove that the grass was not greener, and that it was a good thing I didn't leave my husband for SB1. If you visit The Dirty, a gossip website specifically for players, he is on it. On that site is information that explains how he is known for doing this to many women, too many to list. I may be the only one who has written a book including him and his sliminess. Things with the Vegas chick ended after about three to four weeks. He used her for a place to stay while in Vegas during The Olympia for photo shoots and other work before and after, the same way he used me. Rumor has it she ended up punching him in the face and kicking him out. See, his parents are not well off; they live with his sister and her child in a small apartment in Chicago. When he came home to Chicago, he needed a place to stay, hence using me. Plus, he used visiting his four year old nephew battling cancer as a way to boost his social media following. He has even preyed upon other top male Olympians and athletes to gain their following. He doesn't just play women, he plays men. There is more to my story about SB1 coming up.

In late August, early September, I was devastated after all that had happened between us. Once I figured out he was playing me, my sadness turned into "pissed-offness" and smartness. I was not going to shed anymore tears or energy on this guy; he lied to me. He completely and totally played me and a few of the closet people in my life. I headed to Vegas in late September to work for bodybuilding.com and to compete in The 2012 Bikini Olympia. I had photo shoots booked, and lots of visiting planned with local friends and my fitness family traveling to The Olympia as well. I had no time to dwell on SB1. I had way too many amazing things happening in my life. The only downside of the weekend was that he was supposed to be there by my side for this major event. Instead, I experienced it alone. At this point in my life, I was used to it--being alone. Would you rather be alone during your successes and career highlights, or during your lowest, weakest, most depressing life events? I've been alone for both. I have always had my tribe, my army of angels, both family and friends, who are like family by my side. I'm sure many of you can relate and understand. Family and friends are great, but it's nice to have the support of your significant other, no matter what the event. I am not complaining; just keeping it real. I was alone in my marriage and so many other times throughout my life. I am just grateful for the strength God has given me. I know that in the scheme of things there are bigger problems in this world to complain about.

The Olympia weekend went well. I was honored to grace the stage with the best IFBB Pro competitors in the world. I made it to the top of the sport, the Olympics of bodybuilding, fitness, figure and bikini. Remember when I switched from Fitness America and Ms. Fitness USAs, and how I was so scared I might fail competing in the NPC/IFBB? Well looking back, it feels pretty amazing to see my dreams come true. I remind myself every time I am making a change that it's normal to be afraid and have fears, but I have always succeeded, no matter what I set out to do. I also believe in myself which is half the battle.

I left Vegas and headed back home for a few days. I needed to unpack and repack for New Delhi, India. Bodybuilding.com was sending me to compete in the 2012 Sheru Classic, a professional bodybuilding, figure and bikini competition. My father was born in Pune, India but I had never been to his homeland. Everything about this trip was amazing. I do remember catching my flight from Chicago direct to India and spending about 45 minutes unpacking and repacking my bags in order to make the carry-on bag weight limit. I am not good at packing light! I was a little stressed, figuring out how to get my food for the long flight in my bag with my bikini heels, makeup, and laptop. The airline literally gave me a doily bag. I did it though. I had an entire row to myself which was sweet considering the flight was about fourteen plus hours.

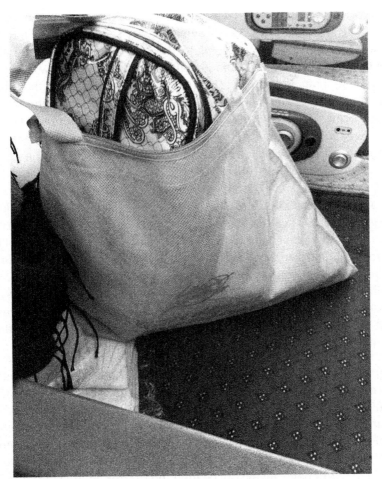

It didn't hold diddly squat! But I made it work.

Upon arrival, each athlete was given a bodyguard. I had arrived before all the other bikini competitors. My first day there, I received a very exciting offer. I was representing bodybuilding.com and working at the same booth with Shashi who owns Unlimited Nutrition, a supplement distributor in India. He is a good friend of the CEO of bodybuilding.com. He asked if I would tour India with Mr. India. They offered to fly me to Mumbai, put me up in The Taj, and pay for my expenses. I, of course, accepted this gracious once-in-a-lifetime opportunity. That entire trip, I know my father was looking down on me, super proud of his little girl, promoting health and fitness in his homeland. While in Delhi, I was taken to a local TV station with four time Mr. Olympia, Jay Cutler and Ms. Figure Olympia, Nicole Wilkins to promote the Sheru Classic on Indian television. Nicole and I even had make-up artists before going on-air. We each had assistants as well, which were a big help with informing us of our schedule and where we needed to be and when. They would also run errands for us, like buying bottled water; being a competitor that is a huge deal, especially when traveling. I packed enough food to get me through the time I would be in New Delhi. I usually freeze my meat in case you wondered and it lasts the entire plane ride.

India is a lot different than America. Traffic is insane. It is non-stop from morning until late at night and people honk their horns frequently. I saw families of three or four on mopeds, something you do not see in the states. Begging children would come up to the cars in the middle of traffic, and some would even perform gymnastic routines in between car lanes. In many areas, one street would be filled with litter, then about a block away you'd see a five-star hotel, shopping, and fine dining, just like in America. The streets were filled with shacks the size of a one car garage where many families lived. I saw women cleaning dishes with buckets of water out on the streets and small children sleeping on hard tables. Seeing this and where my father came from was very emotional for me. How many of you could leave your country to move to another country by yourself, learn another language, and then raise a family? He wanted to find a better life in America, and he did just that. For that, I have always been and will always be grateful for all that I have. It was so difficult coming home from India and not having either parent alive to share the memories with. I want to say "thank you" one more time for all he had provided me with; a beautiful home in an affluent Chicago suburb, a college education, name brand clothing, vacations, a car, and so much more. We in America are spoiled; we have it so good here.

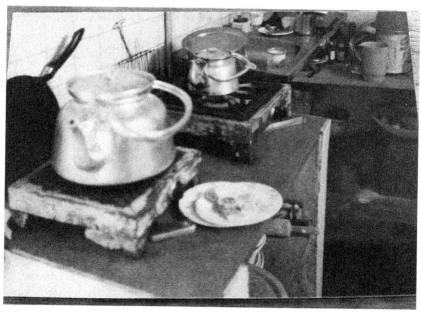

Pictures of my dad's home growing up in India; Kitchen/stove

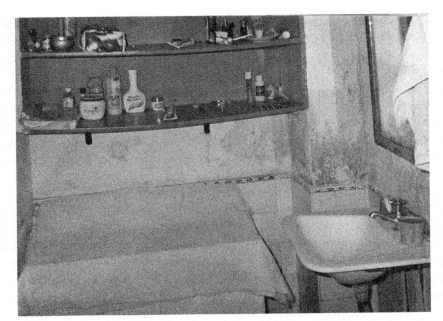

Pictures of my dad's home growing up in India; Bathroom

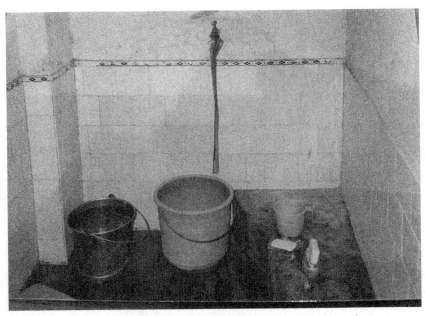

Pictures of my dad's home growing up in India; Shower

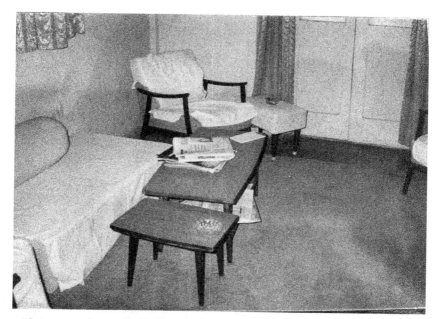

Pictures of my dad's home growing up in India; Living Room

There were thirty plus IFBB Pros that competed in The Sheru in either Bodybuilding, Men's 212, Figure or Bikini. The best in the world were at this show; again, it was another great honor to be one of them. The fans in India are hands down the best in the world. Their enthusiasm and respect for this sport is off the charts. I was the first athlete to go out on stage, and when I did, the entire audience went bananas the entire time I was on stage. They did this for every athlete. The Olympia did not even compare to this. I placed third and won a generous monetary prize. As IFBB Pros, we are awarded money for top placings. Every athlete had a great experience. The day following the show, I had an appearance and then I left for Mumbai with Shashi and his team. They took excellent care of me.

I had a day of rest when I arrived so I was able to sleep in and workout in the posh hotel gym. Shashi even took me shopping and sight-seeing around Mumbai. The following day we had gyms and supplement stores to visit on our road tour. The fans were crazy in a good way, especially at Gold's Gym. We took lots and lots of pictures and signed autographs. Then it was time for me to go home. A 5 day trip turned into an 11 day trip and I am so grateful I was able to see not one but two cities while in India on behalf of bodybuilding.com and Shashi from Unlimited Nutrition. What an experience! It was one I will never forget. It took me 21 days to recover from the jet lag but it was all worth it! So by the time I returned home and fully recovered from these trips, I had completely forgotten about CA1/SB1. I had too many amazing things happening to waste any more time or energy on him.

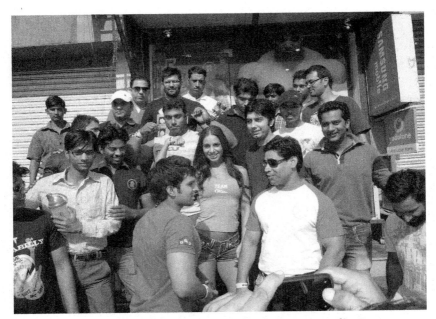

Nicole Moneer 2012, Supplement Store, India Tour

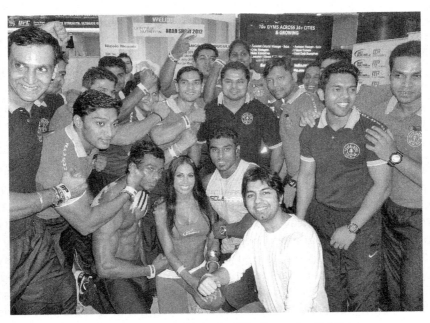

Nicole Moneer, 2012, Gold's Gym, India Tour

I competed in November in Iowa and placed fourth. I had a great end to my 2012 despite my mother's death at the start of the year. On November 29th, I turned the big 4-Oh! I had plans to celebrate that weekend and for weeks to follow. I posted a selfie stating it was my 40th birthday on Facebook. I have three profiles on Facebook; two friend pages and one fan page, so it usually takes me several days to respond and thank everyone for my birthday messages and wall posts. Among the birthday wishes, I received a message from SB2. Yes, moving on...

Chapter 6 - Slimeball #2

"Hey there... Happy belated birthday! I CANNOT believe you are 40.... I'm speechless. I wouldn't have guessed you for 30...wow. Please enlighten me on your secret. I have always enjoyed your smile and personality, but know-ing you are a mature woman just took that admiration to a whole new level! I hope you are doing well. It would be nice to stay in touch my Insta-gram buddy. My cell is (XXX-XXX-XXXX) if you ever feel or have time to chat." - Slimeball #2

Yes, I knew this guy; however, I could not believe he had reached out and con-tacted me. He is one of the head judges for the IFBB. The only conversation we had really had in the past was him providing feedback when on stage, like, "Nicole you need a tighter ass and you need to work on your inner thighs." Hope that makes you giggle. I was not sure if I should respond to his message or not. For one, I was not interested in him at all. I never dated any judge or had any interest in any of them, nor had any judge ever pursued me in the past. I got to the top of the IFBB by myself, with no panties given to anyone. Yes, I did have to say that. Again, I never spoke with SB2 unless it was regarding judges' feedback after competing in a show or replying to comments on social media. I was in a pickle; he was not my type, at least based on looks and my little interaction with him. I wasn't quite sure how to respond, especially since I was competing again one last time in December that year and knew he would probably be at the show. I responded politely back on Facebook with a thank you for his birthday wishes. I did not call nor did I want to.

We messaged back and forth on Facebook for a few days. Then one day he opened up about his ex and her being an addict and so on. He also shared with me that he had been going to counseling for a few years. A man who admits that he needs to work on himself--he totally reeled me in! It was at that point that I thought well, why not give him a chance? He was seven years older than me, he had been through a divorce twice, he was in counseling, and we could easily relate to one another regarding our marriages. He wasn't my type but maybe that was the type I needed to start dating. After a few days of going back and forth on "the book," we took our conversation to the phone. Again, he continued to share more which I found attractive. The plan was for him and me to connect and hang out in Miami. When I arrived, we played it down initially. In the competitor meeting, all judges attend as well. We said hi, hugged, and kept it on the DL. Later, we met up, hung out in the hotel coffee shop, and talked for a few hours. The next day, I competed. One of my guy friends from Chicago came to watch the show since he lives there. When I introduced him to SB2, my friend said, "WTF, Nicole -- he is so not your type!" As I said before, I gave this "man" a chance, especially since he was older.

LL3 was the only other older guy I dated, and only by a year. Since I look young, I attract younger guys, which for me has not been the best thing, I guess.

Before I go on with SB2, I need to mention this important part of my story. I walked into the dressing room backstage for the Miami Pro Show and found a mirror to set up my belongings in front of. A few minutes later, a super cute brunette IFBB Bikini Pro sat down next to me and introduced herself. She asked where I was from and I told her Chicago. She looked at me and said, "Oh, do you know SB1, aka CA1?" She called him by his name, of course. I looked at her and asked how she knew him. She then told me how she and her boyfriend were not doing well and that they (her and SB1) had been talking. I looked her in the eye, and said, "There is a reason you are sitting here next to me today." SB1 had told her he never brought any girls home to meet his parents, except one stripper, and they didn't like her. He wanted her to meet them; he wanted to fly her to visit him out east and vice versa. I said, "Here are pictures of him and me with his dad, sister and nephew. I am not a stripper, and his parents loved me." He was texting her that very moment and I said, "Hey, let's take a selfie together and send it to him." I told her he was a dirt bag, the grass is not always greener, and to stick with her boyfriend, which she did! I told her that everything he had said to her, he said to me and many other girls, specifically brunette bikini competitors. After he received her text of our selfie, he flipped obviously. He told her I was his ex, that I was pissed at him, not to listen to me and that I was making things up, blah blah blah! Either way, God put her next to me to warn her and many others about SB1.

Now back to SB2. I placed 10th out of 22 at the Miami Pro Show, which I was happy with. Personally, I thought this was good, so that when SB2 and I were seen together at the athlete banquet and after-party on Saturday night, none of the other bikini competitors would think there was any favoritism in regards to my placing. I was not dating him for a placing. We had a great time that entire weekend and hung out with other judges, NPC/IFBB staff and competitors, so it wasn't a secret that we were a couple. When I returned home, we talked every day. He then asked me to be his girlfriend and invited me to travel with him to St. Thomas for New Year's Eve. He was flying to the West Coast right before Christmas for his daughter's birthday and my brother was flying into town to celebrate here. Since we had other Christmas plans already in place, we were not able to spend the holiday together. His daughters even picked out my Christmas present though; a Juicy Couture warm-up. My relatives had also thrown me a 40th birthday party in late December since my brother was home in Chicago at that time. My 40th was my first birthday without my mom, so it was wonderful to have over 40 guests celebrate my special day. SB2 lives in Texas. He, of course, paid for my travel expense to St. Thomas, and we met on the East Coast on a connecting flight. The weather was beautiful and we had a great time together celebrating NYE.

Prior to that trip, we had discussed several things regarding us. Actually SB2 liked to plan things as did I. After asking me to be his girlfriend, he expressed an interest in moving forward seriously. He then started planning trips every two weeks to be with one another. So after St. Thomas, our next trip together was to LA for the LA Fit Expo under bodybuilding.com. In December, I had informed my boss that SB2 and I were dating, since they knew him and he too worked for bodybuilding.com. While in St. Thomas, my boss called SB2 and congratulated him on us being a couple. My boss at the time was like a father to me. He then said that our room in LA would be covered while we were in town. SB2 told me all of this. I figured since my boss had called and spoken to him, and was paying for a suite for both of us, then he totally approved of me dating him. While in LA, we were together again for all to see and again had a great time. When I returned home, I had finally finished cleaning my mom's house, almost a year later! That is how much stuff she had. Anyway, SB2 knew that I was finishing matters up on her estate. He texted me, saying that he admired my strength. He also stated that if I needed anything to call, that I was like family and even though he was in important business meetings on and off that week, he would take my call immediately because I was his priority.

Our travel schedule for 2013 looked like this: in the end of January I was traveling to Texas to visit his home and friends. Then in February, he was visiting me for Valentine's weekend and then two weeks later he was paying for my hotel in Ohio since we planned to stay together for the 2013 Arnold Sports Expo. Following that was a competition in Texas that I was scheduled to help him run, then he would come to Chicago again for Easter. In April, SB2 was judging shows in Germany and Rio, so the plan was for me to travel with him to both, for which I had requested time off from my work to attend. We also had discussed my competing. He said that since we were dating, I could not compete, as that would be a conflict with him being the head judge. At that point in my competition career, I was totally fine with that. I had accomplished all I had set out to do with the IFBB. I made it to the top of the sport, coaching myself. If anything, I could judge at the IFBB Pro level, especially since I was an NPC amateur level judge.

While in Texas during my visit at the end of January, we did a lot. He had bought a new puppy which was fun. We worked out, had dinner out with his best friend since age 14 and partner in business, and stayed in one night where I cooked for us. When he dropped me at the airport on Sunday afternoon, my gut had a weird feeling. For some reason, I knew it was the last time I would see him. SB2 was not his usual self. His hug and kiss were pretty weak and quick. He seemed aloof. We talked several times during that week. We talked daily, and then one day he didn't call. He did apologize and said he had a lot going on especially with work, his daughters and his ex-wife. He explained that he was dealing with some problems regarding them. I then had told him, "Your problems are my problems so either way, if you don't' tell me I will feel your stress, and if you do tell me, then at least that way I am aware and can be there for you to lean on if needed." A few days before Valentine's Day, he told me he needed to cut his trip short here while in Chicago since there was a scheduling mix-up with having his daughters that weekend as well. I then started to smell something fishy; he is a bit of a perfectionist and has impeccable scheduling; however, I still gave him the benefit of the doubt. We would talk daily but then he started to blow off calling me. He then informed me that he would not be able to come Valentine's weekend. We were supposed to talk regarding us one night while he was traveling, and he said he would call after a certain time. I never heard from him. Things were starting to become clear.

No one likes not having an answer or to be left hanging... even if the truth hurts.

So I called him at the wee hours of the morning. We finally connected and he broke down on the phone, crying, telling me he could not continue dating me, that he was not in a good place still, and that he needed to be alone. He continued to tell me that his ex-wife blamed him for her suicide attempt. He still had issues about letting others down, and said he felt he had let me down with not being able to visit for Valentine's Day. He said he needed to put his daughters first, especially since it had only been three or four years that he was back in their lives, and needed to work on better relations with them. After that call, I let it be. I did email him asking that he keep his promise of taking care of my hotel at The Arnold, which was less than two weeks away. Rooms for the expo book up a year in advance and my sponsor was flying me out. I certainly did not think it was the professional thing to do to call my boss and say my boyfriend ended things with us so I now need a hotel room. I felt a little like I was in high school with this situation. Now here comes the slimeball part. I notice his interaction on Facebook. Ah, social media; people, the truth always comes out! Why lie and hide it? I swear I should work for the CIA. Anyway, I saw that he was liking another IFBB Bikini Pro's pictures and commenting on them, just like he did mine when we were dating. At that point, once again my sadness turned to anger. I was so pissed! How could this be happening again? He totally lied to me! Here is the other part: he had an affair with this girl when he was married. I somehow was witness to his ex-wife forgiving her at the 2011 Olympia. I always wondered why I witnessed this. When we were in St. Thomas and going forward as we got to know one another better, in the back of my mind I had always wanted to bring up his affair. Since I had one as well, I figured that was another thing we had in common. I never did though.

The next week or so we kept in touch via email regarding hotels while at The Arnold. He said he would pay for a hotel since he had told me to tell bodybuilding.com he was taking care of my hotel, and that I did not need one. He was not having any luck; everything was booked. The night before I flew out to Ohio, we spoke on the phone. He was already in Ohio for the expo and told me that many were without hotel rooms, even people traveling in from Europe to work the event and he was putting out a lot of fires. We agreed that we would keep in contact, and that I would head to his hotel after arriving in to Ohio to see if any rooms opened up later that day. God totally had my back in regards to what happened next. I do enjoy flying to and from The Arnold; the flights are always filled with so many people I know. On the flight out, a gentleman whose seminar I attended a few years back was seated across from me, and he remembered me. We chatted during the flight and when we landed, he and his family offered to give me a ride to my hotel. This gentleman and his family happened to be staying at the same hotel in which SB2 was staying. They kept asking me at what hotel I was staying. I finally came clean and said, "Well this is kind of drama for you." I explained the situation, not in detail like now, but they understood. He said, "Nicole, we have a block of thirty rooms; you can have one of ours as I know we have a cancelation or two." Thank you Lord! So that is exactly what I did. SB2 did keep his part of the promise and sent me the money to cover the room via Paypal that same day.

Every day I was there in Ohio, I ran into SB2. This event is huge with over 175,000 in attendance! The first day there, I saw him at the hotel bar with another athlete who knew him. I spoke to him, and he totally ignored me. Then he kept hanging around the booth I worked during the expo. He would talk to my bosses and the IFBB Bikini Pro that he had an affair with that I mentioned earlier. She too works for bodybuilding.com. I connected with a lot of people over that long week-end, many who last saw SB2 and me together in LA and/or Miami, asking where he was and what had happened. Some even told me things he had said about us that were not true. I come to find out from CEOs and other big wigs that SB2 was the biggest womanizer, a player, and a pig. This was coming from men and women. I couldn't believe nobody had filled me in on this womanizer! If they did though, would I have believed them? I totally had my blinders on. I am not one to gossip and rarely do people gossip to me. That is just how I am. Someone who was a little buzzed even went right up to SB2 and told him off; not because I told her to but because she couldn't believe what he had done to me.

I am totally laughing out loud now about both SB1 and 2. I was looking to retire and move on from the IFBB so I guess my experience with SB2 put a bad taste in my mouth and gave me the impetus to get out even faster. During the time we dated, he filled me in on a lot of things that were shady about the IFBB; the judging, how certain coaches are paid for their athletes' winning, and tons of other drama. For a 47 year old, I was actually turned off by the fact that he got off on all this drama. I am not into any of that. To this day, I am proud that I made it to the top of the IFBB, the most prestigious bodybuilding federation, by myself. I coached myself. I have never taken any drugs to enhance my physique or worn any corsets or squeems to get an hourglass shape. Believe it or not, many girls do in the bikini division. I guess times change since this is the "in" thing to do now. The federation and the fitness industry has a lot of great people, many who are close friends, and the industry has given me many wonderful opportunities. However, like most jobs and industries there are always going to be a few shady people and political stuff.

Upon leaving for the airport, I caught a ride with my good friend, four time Mr. Olympia, Jay Cutler. He knew what was going on since he had seen us together earlier that year. SB2 was in the lobby of our hotel when we left. When we arrived at departures, who was in line in front of us but SB2, and he was with the IFBB Bikini Pro. He escorted her to her flight and then came back to the group I was with. I could not seem to get away from him. I had a bite to eat in the airport with Mr. Olympia Phil Heath, Jay Cutler, and a few others, and of course SB2; he is good friends with Phil. This was weird; he sat at one end of the table, and I at the other. They all knew we were together before and were actually cracking jokes. I was able to laugh along; SB2 on the other hand was not. We finally boarded our flights home. The second SB2 got off the plane, he texted me. I texted him back and basically told him off. I didn't care. I didn't need his approval or liking for any competition placing. I think too many females (and males) are too scared to speak up regarding him for fear of not placing. I am not.

Back to SB1 for a brief bit now; as I mentioned, what matters most to him are "likes" and "followers" on social media. When I see him getting shout-outs on all these profiles saying he is a "good guy," "best man," and to "follow him", I just think, get real. He is SO NOT. He has all of you fooled. At the 2013 Arnold, he ended up hitting on one of my best friend's clients, a brunette bikini competitor, of course. My friend warned her and said, "You know that Nicole is a respectable, good person. He is not a good person and has done some bad stuff to Nicole, so stay away from him," which she did; smart girl. Again, just visit The Dirty. He entered the hotel bar on Saturday night during Arnold weekend while I was talking with his boss and he would not come near us. He knows better. I met his boss through him, of course. There was a group of us now sitting at two tables talking. He had just come from the party where he was hitting on my client's girlfriend. I knew this because my best friend had just texted me all of this. He finally came over to the tables and sat on the complete opposite end from where I was. I was still talking with his boss. SB1 said he was going to walk another female (a co-worker) up to her hotel room and then come back down. After he left the tables, one female fitness model icon at the table asked how his boss and I knew one another. I said, "Through SB1; we dated." She replied, "No wonder why he was acting so weird just now." In the back of my head, I am thinking he knows what he did to me, and he knows he's a true slime ball. People know I am honest and he knew not to come near me. Later that week, I got home and received a text from a well-known male athlete in the industry, an icon, someone who SB1 had conned and actually did video work with. SB1 is masterful at wiggling his way in to well-known male athletes' lives and getting exposure on their social media sties and through their work. This athlete sent me a picture of an Instagram profile with about 400 followers, all hating on SB1. So I was not alone. He had been found out. Too bad his hundreds of thousands of followers didn't know the truth about him. Now mind you, I am not a hater; however, I will warn people about bad people. Maybe that's my mission in life! Anyway, I posted underneath one of the pictures on the profile confirming that all they stated was true; I even tagged SB1. About a minute later, I get a text from him. I never did read it until a few months later. Then the next day I got a text from his boss saying, "Why hate, why post that and why not really leave it to karma?" I replied to his boss via text, "This is not called hating; this is called standing up to a bully. When someone does something wrong, you should tell others to make sure they don't get taken advantage of as well, especially when those people ask you. When is this SB1 going to stop using and playing people? He is a bad person. A perfect example of someone on social media that is fake. He is always saying God bless this and God bless that. He is a dirt bag and not into God at all. I will leave his karma to God, but when asked I will let people know my story, the truth and to proceed with much caution at their own risk."

At 47 years old, SB2, another masterful liar, is a millionaire who had a life that revolved around the NPC/IFBB. If you Google his name though, you will find legal matters regarding harassment with other women. I also found out that he has three daughters and a son. I am guessing he had affairs during his time with his first and second wife. He never told me he had a son. Con artists come into relationships the same way the leave; they come in fast and they leave fast. Women need to know about these types of people. It's good education for women so they know what to look for. I am not sharing my story so people feel bad for me. I feel bad for both Slimeballs really; they are messed up in the head. Regardless of my story and how it comes across to you, I did need SB1 in my life as an important life lesson. Who knows, maybe even a few people reading this now know exactly who I am talking about, will steer clear of him and continue to warn others. As far as SB2, yes I needed him too. It was a perfect exit from the competition scene which is getting toxic. A lot of people, especially girls, want to be me or want what I have in regards to career opportunities, my successes, and more. Do you still want what I have or to be me? Ha! I get a lot of shady, douchey, slimy people that cross my path, and I know I will for years to come. So if you ever question my armor, this is one reason why I have my walls up to so many people that are not privy to have a front row seat in my life.

Chapter 7 - Life Lesson #6 aka LL6

"It is sometimes a disconcerting truth for many Christians that even though we belong to God through faith in Christ, we still seem to experience the same problems that plagued us before we were saved. We often become discouraged and bogged down in life's cares. The fact that both the Old and New Testaments address this problem the same way indicates that God knows problems and worries are inevitable in this life. Thankfully, He has given us the same solution He gave in both Psalms and Peter's letter. 'Cast your cares on the LORD and he will sustain you; he will never let the righteous fall' (Psalm 55:22), and 'Cast all your anxiety on him because he cares for you' (1 Peter 5:7)." http://www.gotquestions.org/turn-over-to-God.html#ixzz3LyCjCE18

Back in Chicago after the 2013 Arnold, I was able to focus on myself again. However, during March, April, and May, I saw posts on social media of SB2 and his new girlfriend. I did delete and block him; however, I would see her posts. They traveled to all the spots he had originally planned to travel to with me. In May, they got engaged. Come to find out, she would be his fifth wife. He had lied to me and told me he had been married only twice. One of my best friends, Stacy, said it perfectly: "You dodged a bullet...matrix-style." Yes, I did. So on with my life and book; I have another player to add to my story for your entertainment.

Pain is how I've grown;

...it's when I've been uncomfortable. When I work out, if I feel pain or discomfort, I keep going because I know my muscles are growing. In life, when I feel pain or discomfort, albeit hard, I keep going because I know I'm growing.

In April 2013, a guy at LifeTime Fitness where I work approached me during my workout. We chatted for about 15 minutes about random stuff. It was not an awkward conversation by any means and he was not hitting on me, at least it did not come across that way. We had never spoken before, even though he had been a member for years, so I thought it was odd that he came up to talk to me out of nowhere. Anyway, over the next few months, we started to chat more when at the gym and then in the summer in late July, we ran into one another at the pool and talked for four hours straight. In late August, we were chatting during a workout, and I brought up the topic of volunteering, and how I had wanted to start again. I was planning to feed the homeless that weekend. He was interested and wanted to know more about the event. He also told me how he had volunteered with his father for his church and some of the things they had done over the years. At that point, I was impressed and thought he wasn't just another guy with a smile and a six-pack. I needed to end my work out that day and train a client, so I asked for his email to send the event info on feeding the homeless. I then emailed him later that night. He responded immediately and asked if he could join me. He also asked if he could take me shopping at Whole Foods (my favorite place, so he listened to me during our conversations), have a barbeque at his house, and then head to feeding the homeless together. I accepted his gracious invite.

The next day, I saw him at the gym and he asked what I was doing Friday. Feeding the homeless was on Sunday afternoon. I did not have plans Friday, so he asked if I wanted to do something. That Friday after work he asked if I wanted to go out for dinner, so I picked a place in downtown Chicago. He picked me up, we ate at the restaurant first, and then headed to a bar after for a few drinks and more conversation. It was a great night. I had just signed my IFBB Bikini contract to compete one last time in Prague and then in India, where I would retire. So after our night out, my restaurant choices would be very limited until after October when I was home and retired from competing. That night he told me he had had a crush on me for four or five years, since 2009. He basically knew everything about me, including my bikini titles, and that I was divorced. He told me he had so much respect and admiration for me for many reasons. For one, he knew that I was a "natural" competitor and that he too had spent almost a decade in the gym trying to gain muscle mass naturally. He also was impressed by my resume and all I had accomplished. He then proceeded to say that he believes God brings two good souls together. So from that day forward, we were together every day, at night and on weekends. We had a good time feeding the homeless too. We would work out together after he got off work. Some nights, we would meet at his house after I got off work, cook dinner together and have great conversations. I met his family at their Labor Day party and his closest friends throughout the next month. I took him to The Bears home opener for his birthday, and then we went and visited his sister in the hospital right after the game. She had given birth to his niece on his birthday. We were together every day for a good six to seven weeks.

In October, LL6 started to pull away a bit. I wasn't quite sure what was happening since things between us were going so well. When I approached him on this, he didn't want to discuss it. Shortly after, I left for Prague. He was supposed to go but couldn't with his work schedule. Bodybuilding.com sponsored my airfare and hotel for this trip. While in Prague, SB2 was the head judge; yippee for me! Anyway, I was happy with my placing. I took fifth competing as the only Bikini Pro from the USA against other European IFBB Pros and I won prize money. LL6 and I spoke daily while in Prague via WhatsApp, an instant free messaging app. When I returned he picked me up from the airport and was excited to see me. One of his best friends had told me LL6 missed me a lot right in front of him. I had no clue he did; he never told me he missed me while I was away but admitted it then.

After a quick two days home, I left for The Sheru Classic in Pune, India. Again, it was my father's birth city, so it was bittersweet to be retiring there. The Sheru brothers sponsored my airfare and hotel for this trip. Guess who was the head judge again? Yep, SB2. Again, I placed fifth and walked away with prize money, so I was happy. Again LL6 was not able to fly out with me to India due to his work schedule and again, we spoke everyday via WhatsApp. When I returned, we worked out at a different gym location than where I worked. I had been gone for over two weeks which my social media following knew so I wanted to spend time with LL6 alone at a gym where no one knew me and we wouldn't be interrupted. He got called into work that night so we were not able to hang out after the gym. We did hangout the next day together though. Then the weekend came and I did not hear from him. I ended up going to his house because we were supposed to do dinner together; we had plans to celebrate my retirement from the IFBB. He didn't open the door but answered his phone, and said he needed some space and that he was afraid of getting hurt. So, I let him be.

Looking back to my last bikini/fitness competition and tour overseas, to be honest, I was glad it was done. How many people say they are going to do something and actually do it? I did it and more. I accomplished what I wanted to so why stay in the sport? It was time to move on to the next chapters of my life. I'm often asked why I did not hire someone for training or coaching as an NPC/IFFB competitor. Why would I do that? I have people seeking my expertise to help them look and feel better, naturally. Why would I hire a coach just to place higher or have a coach take my money for no reason? Truth be told, many hire a coach and never use their workout or nutrition plans; they solely use the coach's name in hopes of winning. People will pay whatever price and do unethical things as well to get to the top. Their egos matter more than anything. I have integrity and I have to say, I know I am among a small group who made it to the top early on without coaches which has inspired many to do the same themselves. Most of the people you see at the top of this sport or winning pro shows are managed or coached. I wasn't expecting to win on this tour; I just wanted to end my IFBB Pro career with a bang! It felt great to compete these last two times in Prague and Pune, India my dad's birth city but again, it was bittersweet! I did not get exposed to the shady side of some people in the IFBB federation until the end. The more I saw, the more turned off I became. In the end, I was extremely happy with my decision to retire. I did not know how bad it really was and is getting. In 2001, I started because of my passion for the stage and performing as did so many. The more I accomplished and climbed the ladder, the more I earned it. No one handed me anything. I definitely met a lot of the right and wrong people along the way, which all helped me in my journey. It took me years to get from A to Z. Today's competitors want it instantly, especially with generation Y. Most aren't willing to work hard. People compete for various reasons, but many of which have to do with the "ego." Some have no clue how much the sport has changed over the last decade; it definitely has an evil side. There are great people in the sport; however, there always will be a dark side as well.

I did what I wanted to do and then some. By creating vision boards and writing yearly goal lists, I made my life happen. How many people can say they did all they set out to do? I know there are many of you reading this that have, can or will. I know there are many of you that have the potential to; you just need to believe in yourself. I finished in this sport where my dad started his life; his birth city. Pretty cool, eh? My dream of world travel for competitions and working other international fitness events was another seed I had planted in my head. Like I teach my clients all the time, dream it; become it.

In early to mid-November, two weeks' time went by and LL6 would text me daily or speak with me at the gym. He asked me out a few times in those two weeks and I was busy each time. Finally, one night he asked if I was free for dinner. We went to Whole Foods, got groceries and cooked at his house. We had some wine and good conversation as well, and had a great night, or so I thought. Then I didn't hear from him again. I left him alone still; I did not want to force him. His best friend from the gym, who most people know as the Ten O'clock News, aka "The King of Gossip", approached me and asked if LL6 and I had been hanging out. I told him yes. He told me that LL6 said we weren't. I was like, "Hmmm, that's weird. We were just together at his house for dinner a few nights ago, and we talk daily." He opened up and stated that LL6 often does this to girls--gives them the runaround; that basically he got what he wanted from me and he was done with me. This was not my first conversation with "The King of Gossip". I knew he was being genuine and looking out for my best interest based on previous conversations with him.

Here I was, wondering if I had been played again. I was not a happy camper. I had a ton of my belongings at LL6's house since we were pretty much living together and with each other daily, especially at night after work. If I asked LL6 to bring me any of my belongings, he wouldn't. He wanted to "hold on" to me and not "let me go," you know what I'm saying? It was strange and pretty controlling on his part. So I waited outside his house for him one night. It sounds psycho but oh no, it wasn't; he had issues with closure or at least me ending things. When he came home, I went inside and grabbed all of my belongings. Then I proceeded to tell him off and that I had figured him out. He was not nice to me at this point. Why would he be? I was telling him off. I took my belongings and left.

He did not come to the gym the next day, my place of work, which was a good thing. The following day though, he did. He made a scene at my work in front of members, claiming I had taken something of his (drugs, which will come into play later) and that he wanted it back. I did not know what he was talking about, nor did I take anything. I had to ask my boss to approach him and tell him to leave me alone at my place of employment, which he did. We didn't talk for a few days. Then I started to get texts from him being nice, asking how I was, and so on. It was Thanksgiving week and my birthday week, which are harder now with my mom being gone. He kept texting me, and I would not reply. Finally, on Thanksgiving I did, and on my birthday. I asked why he was texting me. He started to tell me via text that he has a hard time expressing his emotions, that he liked me too much, and that he was scared. Many of you may think, "Nicole you are such sucker!" Maybe I am! But I like to give people the benefit of the doubt and I too had been in his shoes where it took me awhile to trust again after being burned. Plus, I had been with other guys who had felt like he did. I guess you could say I was being compassionate, especially since I was older than him and more experienced in relationships and life.

On my birthday night, we were together and then he got all funny on me again. I told him I needed more, and if he couldn't give me what I needed, then we needed to end things. I then told him all about SB1 and SB2, and how I thought he was a SB3 (maybe he is; still trying to figure this one out) and that is why I reacted the way I had. He didn't seem to understand until I put my recent dating history out there and in perspective for him. After that discussion, things were great between us. He attended my Luvabulls reunion where 100 of us performed at the half-time. It was his first time ever attending a Chicago Bulls game. He and his best friend had a blast watching us. We went to Christmas parties together, including his family party. We then spent New Year's Eve together in downtown Chicago. I took him shopping beforehand since I know boutiques to shop at for trendy unique clothing and we even got a hotel room to celebrate that night. That weekend, we had dinner with my client and her fiancé. He was aloof all day and pissy when I picked him up to go to their home but we had a good time while there.

By then, we were in 2014, the year of the Polar Vortex. We got pummeled with snow that winter. Outside of being an electrical engineer for his father's company, LL6 also plowed snow for their tenants. If we got hit with a snow storm, he was often busy plowing on weekends and even some weekdays. It wasn't until mid-late January that everything started to make sense to me. He went to New Orleans with a childhood friend to see Dave Matthews; he is an avid fan. We talked every day and night while he was there over the weekend. He even kept me on the phone one night. He wanted me to walk him home from the casino and put him to sleep in his hotel bed, which I did. When he came back in town, I did not hear from him. That night I caught him in lies about his pot smoking. It had become apparent he had an addiction, not just one but two chemical dependencies. I was aware before of his use but didn't realize how frequent it was until then. Even though he wanted me to get high with him I refused; I haven't in over twenty years, since my college days. I didn't realize until that point that all the times he was pulling away was to booze it up and get high. He had been hiding both from me and making up lies--good ones at that--as to why he would distance himself from me. I drink alcohol on rare occasions and the times when we did drink together, we had a lot of fun. Plus, smoking pot doesn't really fly with my holistic healthy image. After I busted him lying, as usual, he knew he had screwed up again with me and was doing anything to get me back. Addicts are masterful liars, and they excel in manipulating people too. This is something that you will not understand unless you have been exposed to an addict or experience life with an addict yourself.

On Friday, January 24th, 2014, I went to my first Reiki appointment, a triad. I had always wanted to do it. It is a physical, spiritual, mental, and emotional healing. I had told them about my parents' deaths, my divorce, some hip pain I was having and that I had missed my period a year ago in May for about 1.5 months due to stress at work. I had too many clients and had to tell people that no, I did not have availability to train them, which for me at that time was stressful. After the session, the practitioner said my mom was present and that she was very proud of me. She also told me I had very good energy. They suggested I get tested to see if I was premenopausal. I said, "No way, do not tell me that." At the very end of my session with them, I gave them a tip and picked a fortune from their bowl. Here is what the fortune said: "BIRTH." I was like, "Huh?" thinking I was not able to not have children at that point in my life. I said, "Why birth? I don't like this fortune, can I put it back and pick again?" They said, "Well it means rebirth with your IFBB career ending, your book, your radio show, and so on." I said, "OK. I like that, thanks." On Monday, I realized I was late getting my period. I was supposed to get it on Friday the 24th and didn't. I am always on time if not a day or two early. I did not stress just yet. I waited to tell LL6 until Thursday that week that I was late getting my period. My gut was telling me I was pregnant, but again I could have been wrong. Women's intuition; I got a lot of it, especially after age 40. After I told him, he flipped out and asked that I get a pregnancy test immediately. I said, "Let me wait until the weekend. Who knows? I may get it (my period) before then." On Friday, I had lunch at an Asian restaurant with a close girlfriend and we opened our fortune cookies at the end of our meal. This time my fortune read, "A package of value will soon arrive." At this point, I was smiling and freaking out, wondering what was going on. My girlfriend knew nothing at the time. I hadn't told anyone besides LL6. Was this my mother talking to me, telling me I was pregnant?

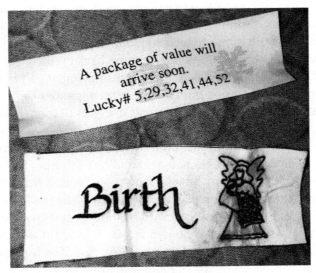

My Fortunes!

So over the weekend, LL6 bought me the test and I took it. At 41 years of age, this was the first ever pregnancy test I had taken. I had to phone a friend to make sure I was reading the result correctly. I had a vertical line and the horizontal line was faint. I texted her a picture and she, a mother of two, texted me, "Congrats, you look like you are pregnant." Literally, I was smiling from ear-to-ear when I read the result. I had always wanted children, but didn't think I could get pregnant. Even though LL6 and I were not married, I knew I wanted this child. I retook the test again on Sunday morning to make sure and again it was positive. It was Super Bowl Sunday and I remember the day well. I drove to LL6's house. He had a few friends over. We hung out alone in his bedroom for a good hour or more. He asked if I was going to keep it and I said yes. He said he didn't want it and that it would ruin his life. He wanted me to get an abortion. I said, "Abortion never crossed my mind. You decide what you want to do and if you want to be a part of this child's life." I knew God had given me this gift but LL6 didn't see it that way. He said if I kept it, he'd be forced to do something he didn't want to do. He didn't want to change his "lifestyle" of partying and not having any responsibility outside of this work.

> *"The mentality and behavior of drug addicts and alcoholics is wholly irrational until you understand that they are completely powerless over their addiction and unless they have structured help, they have no hope." - Russell Brand*

We lay in bed together, and he held me close with his hands over my belly. After an hour, I left his house and headed home. This is where I am going to end Life Lesson #6.

> *"At the bottom of every person's dependency, there is always pain. Discovering the pain and healing it is an essential step in ending dependency." - Chris Prentiss*

I had been off the pill since 2006 and I never got pregnant with my ex-husband. I knew I was meant to have this child with LL6. It's funny, I received some very hurtful, inappropriate texts, phone calls, comments, and Facebook messages, and heard rumors from so many when I went public with my pregnancy in April of 2014. Yes, we received a lot of love regarding our baby-on-the-way; however, I received some not so nice words from a few people that really stung. Many assumed I had never wanted kids; wrong. Many assumed I was too busy in my career and life to have kids; wrong. Many assumed that I was too selfish; so wrong. I even heard that I didn't want to ruin my body by having kids! Wrong again! People also told me though they were glad I finally decided to have a baby and that I had been missing out. Here is the thing: most of these people were not close friends. They knew nothing about me, my personal life, or my marital/dating status, yet they had the audacity to assume and tell me all of this. Here's a tip from me: all the above comments are inappropriate no matter what your relationship is with people.

What happened during my pregnancy, labor, delivery, and postpartum is still too raw for me to share publicly. In book two, I will share how my story unfolds with LL6, and I will include my pregnancy journey, birth story, postpartum along with nutrition and recipes. Nutrition does matter in preconception, pregnancy and postpartum!

"The smarter the woman is, the more difficult it is for her to find the right man." - Oprah Winfrey

Chapter 8 - The Greatest Life Lesson of All- My Relationship With My Father

"Life becomes easier when you learn to accept an apology you never got." - Robert Beault

My Brother Anonymous and I recently had a conversation. We are both divorced; we are both successful in our careers, but not in our relationships. We learned a lot from our parents, both good and bad. We learned many unhealthy behaviors and we also chose partners over and over again who were emotionally, mentally, or physically abusive, much like our father. Reflecting back, I can see and am more aware of how much we as children mimic our parents and how we choose partners that are like them. There is a book out there called Repetitive Relationship Syndrome that proposes that you know better, but you just get stuck in the same cycle. How many of you can relate? My Brother Anonymous and I both have gone down the same path, I sooner than he. Women mature more quickly than men, right? Don't throw eggs at me. Anyway, I started detoxing physically, emotionally and mentally in 2006 and have been doing so ever since. God became a part of my life in my late thirties, early forties. I enjoy Moody Radio with Tony Evans, Joyce Meyers on YouTube and Facebook, the Miles A Minute App with Miles McPherson which my brother turned me on to and I attend church on occasion. Spirituality is not always equated with going to church though. My brother started to follow in my foot steps in his early to mid-forties. He now visits with holistic doctors. God is a big part of his life now and he has been going to a counselor on and off. I am very proud of him and enjoy the conversations we have.

In our family of origin, we saw how much our mother loved us and how she was always there for us, especially when our father was nowhere to be found. However, I saw my mom take abuse from my father; the silent treatments or trying to control her since he was the breadwinner by holding money over her head. It was always either my mom, my brother and I or my mom and I when my brother went off to college. We rarely did things as a family. We maybe had Sunday dinners and parties here and there but not consistently. My mom was comfortable. She was passive. She never did anything. My parents were married for thirty years and most of those years they spent being miserable and living separate lives. In my marriage, I did nothing; we too lived like roommates instead of life partners. I didn't have the tools. Now I do and I also know where to turn for more resources with God in my life, knowing He has a plan for us all, and that when things get horrible, all you can do is trust Him. I am more confident now with the tools Glory gave me and putting my faith in God. I now know how to set boundaries. I am not afraid anymore nor will I be bullied. No relationship is perfect. I control my happiness. I need to stand up for me and so do you. If I don't let my partner and the people in my circle know what I will and will not tolerate, I am the one to blame. We all have our own breaking point.

So here I am, pregnant with child on a new journey called parenthood, potentially going at it alone as a single mother, with a father who's an addict with not one but two chemical dependencies. Either way, it is not at all what I pictured and it's pretty scary! Isn't that life? God's plan? His way; not our way. Hmmm, here I am practically reliving my marriage. Since I'm pregnant now, I can't just walk away this time or maybe I can. Maybe God put me here so this time around I don't quit. Is there something God wants me to overcome? Or maybe God wants me to give it all to Him, to have trust, to believe and have faith? Stay tuned for book two to see how the rest of this part of my story unfolds.

CLIENT TESTIMONIALS

Nicole Moneer helped me tremendously by advising me on nutrition and workouts. I lost 25 pounds and 4 inches in my waist as a result of her guidance and insight. Before I started working with Nicole, I struggled for more than 10 years to lose weight. I also struggled with heartburn and a variety of other physical ailments. Her guidance on eating real food and taking proper supplementation has cured my heartburn and restored my energy levels. I went from a 37 inch waist to a 33 inch waist. Today, my whole family eats differently because they have seen the positive changes in me. I will forever be grateful to Nicole for changing the direction of my life by improving my health. - SCOTT B., ONLINE CLIENT

My time with Nicole has been above and beyond my expectations. I thought I would sign up with Nicole, she would show me a lot of different work outs, I'd get her opinions on different foods and supplements and that would be it. She taught me way more than I could've imagined!

Nicole is teaching me different work outs every time we meet, whether it's lifting weights or doing Pilates Reformer. Nicole reminded me about the importance of yoga (I used to do yoga years ago). Next thing I know we're meeting at a hot yoga studio!

I had been working out five days per week. Two days I would take weight lifting classes and the other three I would use resistance bands, yoga balls, body bars, free weights, and just do my own work out. I was getting bored. I wanted to learn more about what I could do differently with work outs, different ideas for food and what kind of supplements to take. I knew from taking Nicole's "Strictly Strength" class at LifeTime Fitness that I wanted her as my personal trainer. Nicole would mention things over the microphone during class and I would think "this girl knows what she's talking about." I want her as my trainer!

We met twice a week. Once for PT (weights, resistance, etc.) and once for Pilates reformer. Nicole started me on supplements a few weeks after I started with her which was in July 2012. I read a lot of info about supplements because I have a desire to reach optimum health. She also suggested I take a saliva test which reveals information about how my adrenal glands are functioning since she said my symptoms were leaning towards an adrenal issue. I took the test and the results told her what supplement would help support my adrenal glands. I am taking the supplements she recommended and following a nutrition plan she devised for me. Both have helped me a lot! She gave me a lot of options for foods and recipes. I was so excited because I was so bored with the same foods. Nicole told me about the Andi chart at Whole Foods that lists all the nutrients in the vegetables and fruits that they carry. It was amazing! I took pictures of it for my records. She asked me if I had ever eaten kale and I said no. That day after I met her I went straight to Whole Foods and bought kale. Now I love kale and kale chips! This is just one of the many things Nicole has introduced me to.

I had some changes that I knew I had to make. I used to drink a venti Americano (espresso) from Starbucks with a splash of heavy whipped cream, NO sugar, NO sweeteners. I would make this stop at Starbucks every morning! When Nicole recommended supplements to me one of them was a greens drink. She gave me a sample of it. To my surprise, I loved it! I decided I would wean myself off the espresso and drink the greens drink instead. It took less than two weeks to wean myself off my usual Starbucks. Every night I would make dinner for my family and myself. I would love to have one or two glasses of Chardonnay with my dinner. I knew I'd have to cut way back on that. I decided to only have wine on Friday and Saturday nights. Now, I typically only have one or two glasses of wine on Saturday night. Some weekends I don't have any. It's not a big deal to me anymore. Sometimes now since I don't really drink it that much I get headaches from it by the time I'm about to go to bed. Alcohol can interrupt your sleep which was one of my other issues. Now I don't have to deal with that. It's hard on my liver and losing sleep just isn't worth it. I have more energy from cutting the wine and I don't need the caffeine from the espresso the next morning. I started feeling better and better as weeks went on.

Eczema is one condition that I'm still working on. I've adjusted my supplements to try and help with this issue. Nicole told me it is internal. She recommended I get a food and allergy test. I am so happy I did this test. It has helped me tremendously with adjusting my diet and gave me relief regarding chronic problems.

Nicole educated me on detoxes that I could do to help prevent illness and get rid of bacteria and fungus. Everyone has an overgrowth of fungus in their body, especially if you drink regularly, eat sugar and starchy processed carbs regularly, and have been on antibiotics or other prescription drugs. She taught me the importance of your gut. She introduced me to oil pulling. I do this every morning now when I wake up. When she asked me if I had ever heard of it, my eyes lit up and I said, "What's that?" with eagerness to learn all about it. The other detox is the clay which helps clean out your intestines. We bought the clay when we went on a "colonic" date! Another one of Nicole's recommendations for living a lifestyle of prevention.

Nicole also asked me if my doctor was a naturopathic doctor. I said, "No, she's a primary care physician." I talked to my cousin, Shannon, about the supplements I was taking. She ended up referring me to her Naturopathic doctor who I have been going to since January 2013. This experience I had with Nicole led me to a huge decision. I decided to go back to college and study integrative health. I will start a master's program in either Naturopathic Medicine, Oriental Medicine or Acupuncture. I'll figure it out soon but I'm so happy that I am surrounded by like-minded people now and for this new chapter in my life!

Nicole has inspired me to "make my life happen" as she said it. Another thing that always sticks in my mind is Nicole saying "Why not?!" I feel like Nicole has helped me build more confidence to really go for what I want. Before I hired Nicole, I was stuck in my same old routine. Even though people would give me a lot of credit for working out so much, there is so much more to health than "steel and sweat" as Nicole would say. In our first consultation, Nicole pointed out that we need to pay attention to what is happening on the inside of our bodies (our gut), not just the outside. We also talked about how my goal is to reach optimum health and be a role model of health for my 10 year old daughter. It means the world to me to influence my little girl to live a healthy lifestyle. Nicole also taught me how emotions will affect our health. We hold on to toxins in our bodies via emotions. These emotions can show up as chronic pain or disease and pose problems with various organs. I really appreciate Nicole's lifestyle. I feel like we get each other. Most people would look at us like we're crazy for carrying food in our purses, so we don't have to resort to making bad choices by eating out since most places do not serve antibiotic hormone free meats or organic vegetables and fruits.

I told Nicole that it is so refreshing to have her as not only my personal trainer and life coach, but now a great friend in my life. I thought I was going to hire Nicole as my trainer and learn some new workouts, which I did but I got so much more in the end. I found a desire for what I am so passionate about; what goes on inside our bodies, what we are putting in and on our bodies, and how we can change and prevent disease. I am so blessed to have Nicole in my life. She has led me to change my life in a positive way. It's not that it wasn't positive; I was just in a standstill. Nicole is my angel! - MAUREEN B., CLIENT

I had an unhealthy relationship with food going from one extreme to another; starving and binging. I used to work out just so I can eat whatever I wanted. Eventually, I would get too busy or get tired of working out and eating to my heart's content would catch up with me. I'd gain weight and be unhappy about how I looked and work out like crazy (sometimes as much as 2-3 hours/day) to lose the weight. Every two to three years, my weight would fluctuate from 105 lbs. to 135 lbs. After having two children, injuring my knee, and suffering from severe migraines, the years of yo-yo dieting finally caught up with me. I reached my heaviest weight at 160 lbs. I've always been very active but lost interest in doing things that I enjoyed after gaining so much weight. I had my blood work done and my fasting glucose, triglyceride, cholesterol and blood pressure were all elevated. I had a hard time walking up the stairs without shortness of breath and didn't have the energy to play with my kids. This was a HUGE wake-up call for me. My doctor said I needed to start taking medications to keep my levels normal but I knew I didn't want to start taking them at such a young age and had to do something about it.

I joined a gym and worked out regularly and completely changed my eating habits. I used to do 2-3 hours of cardio to lose weight but I've learned to workout smarter and not spend hours in the gym, thanks. I eliminated processed/ artificial foods and started eating smaller frequent meals. After working out about an hour a day, six days a week and eating clean, I was able to lose 42 lbs. in 24 weeks.

I began training with Nicole January 2013. She helped me to sculpt my body and coached me with nutrition, posing and every aspect of competing including suit selection, hair, make-up, tan, etc. She developed a nutrition plan for me to follow and kept tweaking every couple of weeks until the day of the competition. She kept me motivated and inspired me during my transformation journey, especially during the times I began doubting myself and wondering what I got myself into. During our first session, I had mentioned to Nicole that I was unhappy about how my abs looked and thought about getting laser treatment/ surgery to flatten and smooth them out. She strongly advised against it and told me that working out and changing my diet alone would take care of it. Sure enough, after working hard for ten weeks, she was right! After having two children, I was able to have flat abs and got into the best shape of my life. At 40, I'm more fit now than in my 20s. I now have a healthy relationship with food and practice what I preach.

It's important to make your health a priority and set a good example for your family. During my transformation journey, my husband also lost 30 lbs. with eating clean and weight training. Not only was this a physical transformation, but a mental one as well. I've become more positive, optimistic, confident and a happier person. _- NANCY K., CLIENT_

Growing up I was very active. I was a third overall state gymnast, ran track, dove for my high school, played softball and was a Division I soccer player. I have always had an athletic body, but never really focused on building lean, toned muscle. After college, and three knee surgeries, I started my professional career in IT for one of the Big Four consulting firms. I eagerly entertained clients and worked long, stressful days, focusing on doing a good job for my company, completely neglecting my body, health and overall wellbeing. Over the course of 12 years, I have gained weight and yo-yoed between 30-40 pounds, slowly eating away at the confidence I received from my professional life.

My fitness journey began when my husband asked if I would actually go to the gym if we got a membership to Lifetime Fitness. Knowing that it was three times the cost of our current membership and being conscious of our finances, I said yes with reservations. After about one month of running on the treadmill for twenty minutes, three times per week, completely avoiding weights and seeing no results, I finally signed up for an assessment with the head of the Personal Training Department. I shamefully stepped on the scale, and then sat down with him to talk about goals. He actually made me commit to doing something about the way I felt, then threw the icing on the cake... my husband had signed up for personal training, so he could get in better shape than me! I didn't realize it at the time, but that was the kick in the butt that I needed to spark the competitor in me to make a change. We set a goal to lose twenty pounds in five months.

I agreed to sign up for personal training sessions, but under one condition; that I would get a female trainer that knew how to get results, especially for athletes, like me, that didn't want to bulk up. Little did I know at that moment that my one wish was about to be granted. Nicole Moneer, who is an IFBB Bikini Pro, bodybuilding.com athlete, and an NASM Certified Personal Trainer was available to take on another client! I cannot begin to say enough positive things about Nicole and all that she has taught me. Her best skill is that she truly understands how to read her clients, even when they have no idea what they're talking about or asking for! I'll never forget my first session with her; walking dumbbell lunges and pushups on a barbell. I thought I was in decent shape, but she quickly proved to me that I needed to work a lot harder to achieve my goal. I couldn't walk for four days without several muscles feeling some kind of pain; that was November 22, 2011. Since then Nicole and I have been lifting weights twice per week and training on the Pilates Reformer once per week. I also work out on my own, doing cardio and weights. So far, there have been two big moments that have given me the motivation to continue: first, snow skiing with no knee pain. For those of you who have bad knees, you know the kind of pain I'm talking about, and after five hours of non-stop skiing, I felt no pain. I couldn't believe that I could ski two days in a row for the first time in 16 years! Second: stepping on the scale and seeing ten less pounds and three less inches on my waist. Yay... finally, results! And I don't feel bulky! In fact, I have actually realized that my fear of weights making me bulky was a bunch of bologna. Another important note that I need to mention is that Nicole had suggested a meal plan from the start in November but I said no. After a month of working out with her and not seeing results though, I decided to give the meal plan a try. Not only did I drop ten pounds in one month, but I also ended up finding foods that I love so I am able to make it a lifestyle while keeping the weight off. My trainer, Nicole, knows best, and she would always say, "Nutrition is king. Sweat and steel alone will not help in reaching your fitness and health goals. You must do all three together, consistently."

I began to notice the biggest changes when I started Nicole's meal and supplement plan. Nicole meticulously created a personalized plan based on my Stress and Resilience Test and fitness goals, then monitored my progress, offering suggestions and coaching along the way to keep me on track. The Stress and Resilience Test was worth it since it showed that working out later at night was better for me and it also suggested supplements to help balance out my cortisol levels. I had to remove several things from my daily intake, but the results were unbelievable. I finally have more energy and can stay up past 10:30 pm on date night! Seems sad for a 32 year old, but previously I was so drained from work that I usually ended up falling asleep in the middle of the movie. The best part is that I don't feel deprived, even when I'm tempted with my favorite foods; chips and salsa.

As of February 2012, I still had a long way to go but I then decided to add a new goal. I asked Nicole for her professional advice on whether or not she thought I had what it took to compete in an NPC Bikini competition like she does. Nicole said, "You can do anything you set your mind to. If you believe it and want it then yes, that is a great goal for you!" So with Nicole's help, the support of my loving husband and the wonderful staff at Lifetime, I started a new journey of transforming my body to be on stage in a bikini.

With a new goal set, my meal and supplement plans changed as did my time in the gym. I went from four days to six days per week, willingly. So my new outline consisted of working out with Nicole twice per week, and then four days on my own. She always mixed it up, from weights to High Intensity Interval Training to TRX suspension training to battle ropes, she always kept my body and mind guessing. I enjoyed how she continually challenged me in so many ways. In fact, since our start in November, we never did a single workout twice! I consistently did at least four days of cardio for forty minutes, switching between Zone 2 some days to Zone 3 and 4 other days. I also hit the weights at least three of the other days on my own for a total of five times per week. The Pilates Reformer class was a great compliment to my program; my workouts were getting more intense so it was great to be able to de-stress and stretch, which really helped with my flexibility and core strength.

From February through May my weight continued to drop. I bought new workout clothes since everything was falling off me and I was now able to fit into pants I hadn't worn in years. No complaints from me! In May, my husband and I spent two weeks in Europe, and I was concerned I would gain my weight back and fall off track while away. But guess what? Nicole is an expert when it comes to traveling the world and staying on track with your workouts and eating as well. She made several suggestions for foods to pack while traveling and what to order when eating out. She even wrote up hotel room workouts, in case I didn't have access to a gym. I think I only gained about 4-5 lbs. while on this trip. When I returned in late May, we set a date for July 6th to compete in The NPC Chicago Pro-Am. My goal with this show was to transform and push my body to a whole new level. I did that and more. I took third place! In the end, I was down 29 pounds and lost eight inches on my waist and six inches on my hips. The only thing I gained was a healthy new way of life!

In the seven-and-a-half months I worked with Nicole there were many times I mentioned a goal for starting a family with my husband. My husband did not want to have any more children, which upset me greatly. Nicole told me not to give up on my husband or my marriage and to seek counseling with her therapist, Glory. It helped me to really take a look at myself so I could better communicate my needs to my husband and better understand his needs. The counseling proved to be a success! They say timing is everything. A few weeks after I competed in July, my husband and I found out I was pregnant. We were both so happy with this news! I met with Nicole on occasion during my first trimester to help keep me on the right track while pregnant and to continue to add to my workout program. I am due any day now!

I am really proud of my progress, especially when I think back to when I couldn't even do one push up! I give all the credit to Nicole, who stuck by me since the beginning. She wouldn't let me give up and always knew exactly what I needed to hear to re-focus and stay positive. She truly is an inspiration to me in every sense of the word! Training with Nicole was absolutely the single most critical component of achieving my original goal of losing weight, not bulking up, and adopting a healthier lifestyle. Not only is her knowledge of the body and nutrition second to none, but also her ability to understand how my body was progressing when I struggled to see results helped to keep me motivated and focused on continuing to work hard and eventually get results. The support and variety of fitness programs offered at Lifetime make up a well-rounded package that can help anybody achieve any goal. I love the way that the weight lifting combined with Reformer Pilates has shaped my figure and helped me move and feel better overall! Thanks to Nicole for her consistent encouragement, coaching, and constant reminders that I can do anything that I set my mind to. - STACIE K., CLIENT

I met Nicole Moneer when she first became a trainer with Lifetime Fitness in Chicago roughly 8-9 years ago. I remember when I first sat down with her when I was in my early twenties. She talked about meal planning, proper training, and how ideal health goes far beyond the 1-2 hours a day you spend in the gym. She reviewed expectations and spent a good amount of time going over things with me, but I didn't end up signing up at the time and, looking back, I just wasn't ready. I never cooked and didn't have any sense of urgency or motivation to learn how to. I ate fast food (McDonalds, Taco Bell, or Pizza Hut) five or more times a week, and I truly believed that in order to get in shape I needed to work harder and longer. I would do hours of cardio a week without seeing results, and I just felt stuck in a rut.

I struggled with sinus infections, frequent colds and sicknesses since my early teens and well into my mid-twenties. My immune system was never strong enough to fight colds on its own so I was frequently taking prescription medication. I began to pick up on patterns with my body and notice that whenever the seasons changed, I'd end up with an upper respiratory infection - not fun.

At 25, I began to experiment with natural medicine and an acupuncturist who studied both ancient French and Chinese acupuncture. Over time with numerous treatments my immune system got stronger and I no longer need Rx. I would drink plenty of fluids, get eight plus hours of sleep a night, and drink hot tea. Again, I still didn't change the way I ate, so I would still get sick; however, my body was getting strong enough to fight off infections on its own for the first time in my life!

Mid to later twenties, I worked with several different trainers, but I never seemed to "gel" with them. Some recommended fat burners and excessive cardio, and it was just getting tiresome. My workouts continued to get more intense, but each year I was gaining a little bit of weight and my body wasn't changing in the way I'd hoped. To say I was frustrated is an under-statement. I started to learn how to cook, and it probably took me 3-4 years to really finesse a fresh, hot off the grill, yummy chicken breast! I can now say, with confidence, I've mastered it! It took some blood, sweat, and tears to become the good cook I am. I'm a picky eater to begin with, so if I was going to adapt a healthier lifestyle, I knew it was imperative for me to learn how to make food taste good.

Shortly after learning how to cook, I started following Nicole on Facebook and various social media sites. I truly believed in the postings and com-ments she would write on finding balance, proper nutrition, well-being, and happiness in life. I knew in my heart she was someone I wanted to work with. She is far beyond a "personal trainer." Nicole is a genuine soul that takes pride in her work and each and every person that she touches. She is a life coach who has taught me how to find balance in my life with work, health, and relationships, and has helped me through many ups and downs in the time that we've worked together. I feel that she has given me the knowledge and tools to know how to properly fuel my body for life. I love her holistic approach to coaching, which has taught me how to benefit from foods that heal the body from inside out. When I first started follow-ing one of the meal plans she custom designed for me, I was working out less than I had in the past, and yet my body was responding positively - It was mind blowing. I started dropping weight, my abs had more definition than I'd ever seen, I was healthy, and I felt more stable. I didn't experience up and down moodiness because I was eating good quality, wholesome foods. I never felt deprived and I had more energy.

Nicole also helped me achieve a long time goal of competing in a figure competition. This was something I've wanted to do for almost ten years, but I never thought I would be capable of accomplishing. The best part about working with her was she had a plan A, a plan B, and a plan C. What I mean is that she administered plans in stages to help me better prepare. Once the competition was over she had a new custom meal plan ready for me to launch immediately to help reintroduce my body to foods I had not had in a while. The competition was a great experience and I think my big-gest take away was how important it is to properly reintroduce foods back into your system. When you train for months eating organic, hormone free meats, low grains, and healthy fats, and then you over indulge in junk, your body is going to talk back to you; it may be very upset with you! Nicole has *taught me and anyone she works with that food can help heal or destroy you.*

Over this last year I've changed my lifestyle and have adapted a new mindset in how I view food due to Nicole's teachings. I like to compare it to cars. We wouldn't put crap fuel in our cars. Why? Because they would run terribly and likely break down over time. Similarly, why would we put crap food in our bodies? I know what eating healthy feels like and how it feels when I don't, so I choose the first option. Fueling your body with proper food, lots of water, plenty of sleep, and healthy relationships can truly turn back the clock. Once you can find balance with food and exercise, you can let the food work in your favor. In another words, I've always had to "train" with intensity all the time; cardio with every session because my eating was excessive and I would over indulge. My joints ached and it was hard at times to find motivation. One of the first things I told Nicole when we began to meet in November 2012 was "I want to lift and leave." I can now say after working with her for almost two years, with two small shows under my belt, and lots of great cooking recipes from her, I now generally do one to two 30 minute cardio sessions weekly, three to four lifting session, not more than an hour a day in the gym, five days per week and I'm maintaining my current weight and feel great! This is the first time in my 13 years of exercising that I am not killing myself with hours and hours of cardio.

I'm grateful and blessed to have met Nicole and to have had the opportunity to work with her. As I've turned 30 in June, I look forward to a healthier lifestyle, and to continue to learn and grow from the best! Love you booty by Nicky! Thank you from all my heart on everything you've taught me and your continued support. - EMILIE A., CLIENT

I met Nicole around December of 2011 when joining Lifetime Fitness in Schaumburg. I had been working out for about four years previous to working with her. Was I in shape? Yes. Did I eat healthy? No; I thought I did but it wasn't healthy for me. So prior to training with Nicole, I was introduced to fitness by a boyfriend. All he showed me was lifting weight in the gym. Due to the fact he started my journey I trusted him. It wasn't until I met Nicole that I started variety in the gym as well as the kitchen. I ate your typical egg whites, chicken breast, broccoli; same old typical cookie cutter diet. Little did I know I was growing allergies from constantly eating the same food. And on top of that, I have food sensitivities that run in the family. Nicole taught me how to rotate my fats and protein and keep variety so that my body made constant progress. She also taught me the importance of eating whole natural food, antibiotic/ hormone free and organic. She

helped me to understand that paying the farmers, not the doctors was key. I was introduced to Nicole by another Lifetime employee that ranted and raved about her expertise in mainstream health/fitness as well as competition prep. As far as diet goes I was a wonderful client, listened well and followed all her advice. With her knowledge I made huge changes and improvements in my body I had never seen before. As we all know, diet is 80% of how we look. We can work out until we're blue in the face and still struggle to see the results we want.

Now, as far as training goes, I had a lot of variety with Nicole. She taught me and guided me the way I needed to be taught. I will admit I was hard headed and was so stuck on training heavy, because it was all I had known previous to working with Nicole. Now she was preparing me for bikini for the NPC Federation. Bikini has a very specific look; lean, tight, curvy, tiny, long muscles-- especially at my size since I'm very short on stage and I appear thicker than other girls with the muscle I carry. When I started with Nicole, I had huge legs and a lot of muscle. I didn't quite understand at first what the judges were looking for. Nicole only tried guiding me in the right direction to get me the look I was supposed to have. Now, it took me several shows to understand and learn my body. Finally, after letting go of my ego and stubborn side, I listened to all she ever told me and stopped lifting weights period. I also run every other day now. I even had to stop working my lower half period for months to get this bulk off. It took lots of hard work to lose muscle. So I threw myself for a major loop.

In addition to all of this, Nicole not only has done all of the above, but has also been a stepping stone to helping me gain a lot more confidence with myself as a whole. When you have a personal trainer you need to only listen to them and be open about everything to be able to make changes and improvement. You cannot let outsiders that have no knowledge ruin that! Keep all your eggs in one basket. So, I finally became independent. I am now solo, meaning single, and have finally found myself and confidence. People don't realize the importance of learning to be alone and finding themselves. I have been in and out of toxic relationships throughout my life. I finally took that chance, and let go of people that weren't adding positivity to my life. I am a very routine person, and have a huge heart, so it is very hard for me to let go of a relationship I've been in for a long time. But by finally letting go and flying away like a bird, I have learned to spread my wings. As Nicole always told me you have to have a relationship with yourself first before anyone else! So true!! How can we focus on us and our dreams, challenges we face in life, and goals when we put so much energy in to a relationship? Nicole opened up my eyes to a lot; I just needed to apply her advice.

Throughout my journey with Nicole, I was so focused on winning my pro card in the beginning and she would always tell me it's not about that. Now I understand why she told me that. Fighting, and having the thick skin that it takes to compete alone is a blessing. Most of all, the journey I have been through and what I have learned through the sport has helped me and guided me to who I am today. I've learned how to love the journey, and am happy to be able to add to my story. I feel that I was brought in this world to inspire. I used to be an overweight, miserable, irresponsible, lazy person. But I have blossomed into a butterfly and learned to love myself from the inside out. No matter what size women are or situation they're in, they need to have faith and keep pushing to reach their goals and dreams!! Women, it hasn't been all peaches and cream for me. I have a very deep journey and have struggled through my past 28 years. My story only continues to grow. I finally get it; it all makes sense now as Nicole tried helping me and explaining things this whole time. I have Nicole to thank for giving me a very special gift and leading me to an amazing life. Love you Nicole! - SAMANTHA S., CLIENT

I initially reached out to Nicole for competition prep. After our first meeting, I knew working with her was going to be different. At that time, I had no idea the impact she would have on my life both inside and outside of the gym.

My husband and I of eight years were going through a very rough time. Although it was difficult, I shared our story with Nicole. Immediately her heart opened up and she was able to empathize with me. I instantly felt that she understood me as she shared her life experiences with me and gave me advice. This was exactly what I needed to hear at a really dark and difficult period in my life.

We discussed relationships and the importance of taking care of a marriage. She also recommended a really compassionate relationship therapist in my area. The best choice I made was that first appointment with the therapist. I learned a great deal about myself as an individual, and as a wife. I will never forget the words Nicole told me: "Love is a choice." She couldn't have been more correct. I made the choice to work on my marriage and it is now better than ever. A great deal of this success was due to her encouragement and advice.

Nicole is the most genuine and compassionate person you can hope to cross paths with. She truly cares about her clients inside and outside of the gym. She has been a leader and an inspiration for me in many facets of life. I am truly blessed to be able to call her my "coach." - HEATHER M., CLIENT

I've worked with Nicole for nine months, twice a week in one-on-one sessions. I knew of her from just being a member at Lifetime Fitness, where she was a trainer and taught some classes I took. For several years, I admired her posts on social media, in which she emphasized the importance of proper nutrition as a form of preventative medicine, as well as the power it can have in healing chronic disease and illness. The results of some of her clients were really impressive. I saw that she worked with clients on healing their bodies from the inside out, training smarter and not harder. These ladies looked amazing and more importantly, they said how great they felt.

I have been a frequent gym-goer for 13 years, working out 5 days a week very consistently. Although my diet was much healthier than the average person, I definitely wasn't eating clean consistently and drank wine with friends during our weekly gatherings. After I had my first child, I got back to the gym and my pre-pregnancy body pretty quickly, but I decided it was finally time to take it to the next level with my fitness and lifestyle. Nicole was just coming back from her maternity leave, so we were both new moms. I have to admit, I had thought of hiring her in the past, but was a little intimidated by her since she was an IFBB pro bikini athlete. I wasn't sure I'd be as strict with the nutrition as she would suggest. After finally signing up for sessions and meeting with her, I quickly realized that my assumptions of her were completely wrong! She explained that everyone comes to her at a different level and she was the furthest thing from being intimidating. She's easy to talk to, very open and honest, and will be your biggest cheerleader!

Nicole helped me tremendously with cleaning up my diet. Within the first three weeks, I got amazing results following her plan. The fat literally melted off and I lost two pant sizes within a month!! And the best part was that I was doing a lot less cardio — only thirty minutes twice a week! I used to avoid lifting weights, except in group fitness classes. She helped give me confidence in the weight room and now I lift weights five days a week. I love the variety of her workouts and have never repeated the same workout twice. A few events (vacations, weekend getaways) made me fall off track here and there, but with Nicole's guidance, I'm always able to get back into my size 2 pants without the extra bulge. She has also taught me not to beat myself up, and that it's okay to let life happen and get off track sometimes. I tend to be very hard on myself and she has worked with me on that in our sessions.

On another note, when I first started working with Nicole, my daughter had been getting sick with colds on and off. She referred me to someone she had worked with in the past that helped me with detoxing my daughter *and getting her on some good quality supplements. So not only was I getting healthier with Nicole's nutrition plan, but so was my daughter. My husband has also slowly been influenced by my healthy lifestyle. He often lacked energy and felt bloated and sluggish during the day. He signed up to work with Nicole on nutrition and she first got him off of gluten and dairy. He noticed immediate improvement.*

During our sessions, we talked about many things, not just nutrition and exercise. She's really knowledgeable on a lot of subjects, especially when it comes to emotions, communication, and relationships. This is important because people often don't think of their emotional wellbeing as having a connection with being physically and nutritionally fit. However, many times people have underlying issues that hold them back when it comes to starting and maintaining a healthy lifestyle - both inside and outside of the gym. Nicole has been such a positive influence in my life and she's so much more than a trainer to me. She's been a mentor, given me great advice and referrals, and lifted me up when I was feeling discouraged. She's a great example of practicing what she preaches and respects that everyone is on a different journey. Hiring Nicole was one of the best things I could have done for myself and my family! - Melissa S., client

This is why I love my job! To touch other people positively in their professional and personal lives is one of my greatest accomplishments. I have excellent people skills, which I use in my personal training business and in all industries I have worked in. You can be the best at anything, but if your people skills stink, then your business will suffer. Working for Nordstrom, Claire's, Conair, Bally Total Fitness, LifeTime Fitness and bodybuilding.com have given me great experience in people skills and event planning. Even my extracurricular activities as a child have impacted my networking skills today. This is not something you wake up with; you have to work for this. I have become a trustworthy information system for people. When people want something they get in touch with me, and not just regarding fitness and health either. It's a great feeling to know that people trust me with where to go and who to work with regarding almost anything in their life. I built these contacts over many years and trust was created so I don't just turn over names and numbers when asked. People, you need to earn that kind of information yourself. Networking or "friend-working" is huge, and I love being that person for people.

MY ADVICE TO COUPLES (IF YOU WANT IT)

We develop from our struggles. God has put all these Life Lessons, Douchebags and Slimeballs in my life to teach me. In the words of my publisher, I have a Ph.D. in life. People of both sexes and all ages love to be around me. They are inspired from my stories and often come to me for advice. My overachieving nature stems from my father's abandonment and neglect. Because of his harsh criticism, I felt I was never good enough for him. I always sought his approval and the approval of others. Do do do, to get love and get noticed. I was fueled to prove a point by doing what everyone expects of me and more, especially my father. Through my childhood wounding, my personality developed. My life would not have turned out the way it has had things been any different. When I stopped running so hard and giving people power in my life, and finally let God lead me, I started to live in the present moment at peace with myself.

I wouldn't change my divorce with all that God has given to me since. My father's death and my mother's death were gifts as well. God can turn a weapon into peace and a gift for you. It's all perspective and how you look at each life circumstance.

You must love yourself before you can love another.

I learned to accept the dark side of me. I learned to love all of my parts, the good ones and the bad ones. In my later years I've been more open with friends, clients, family and those I dated. Allowing myself to be vulnerable and weak has actually helped me create a stronger bond with most people. That is what true intimacy is; being vulnerable and weak. It has been very difficult but has improved the quality of my life. Soulseeds.com is a great website for more on how to love yourself.

To anyone who takes a vow to be married, "for better or worse" is not to get a divorce but to stay and fight.

Get help, even if you go solo to a counselor, and if you don't have money talk with your pastor. Your partner may or may not follow and that's OK. Work on yourself and everything else will fall into place. In any relationship, two people need to stay and fight. Usually one wants to work and the other does not, especially in this day and age. Most quit; it's what many of us are taught. Marriage is like flies on a screen door. You got some waiting to get in and then you got some waiting to get out. LL4 and I both agreed that we learned some great tools at the Retrouvaille retreat. In marriage, both people have feelings that matter; this is the key factor. Most feelings are being discounted, most do not know how to communicate their feelings and most are too ashamed or embarrassed to share their emotions and past hurts. Nothing in life teaches us this; we need schools for our emotions. Oprah, are you reading this? I hope so. Adults are hurt children; we all have pain that stems from our younger years, whether we admit it or not and it has a profound impact on our adult relationships. Everybody just wants to be loved, appreciated and respected. Why is this so hard?

"The only way a relationship will last is if you see it as a place you go to give, not a place that you go to take." - Anthony Robbins

Give your partner more love, more appreciation and more respect.

Everything happened the way it needed to be. I am better, not bitter and I get to share my story which might just help someone else. Many have called me for advice because they too ended up where I did; lost, having an affair. The first questions I ask anyone who comes to me are "What is going on with you? What are you unhappy about? What needs of yours aren't being met? What more could you do? Are you putting your energy into your partner and your marriage or outside into someone or something else? How have you contributed to the demise of your relationship at this point?" Until you change, nothing will change. Changing means you have to change your despondence. Sometimes the hardest thing to do is the right thing to do. I shouldn't have had an affair; I should have just left LL4, period! Maybe he would have come running after me or maybe he wouldn't have. It takes a lot of strength to just walk away from someone and say I need to be a priority in this relationship, I can't live like this. I was weak. I am human, and I sinned just like you.

What you do to yourself, you do to your spouse.

You better know who you're marrying because they will have the greatest influence on you over anyone else. Their problems become your problems. Everyone has problems, but the question is, how do you and your spouse handle problems and do you admit or deny? The first three to six months you don't really know them, so you're infatuated. Date at least a year so you can see them through all their seasons.

If you're married, you must be on the same team.

Seek counsel in your spouse. Make heated discussions a win-win. It's OK to ask for a timeout; that way things don't get too heated. You can always regroup later. Couples typically fight because of neglect or feeling threatened. Try your best to listen to your partner. More often than not they are not nagging; their needs just aren't being met. Listen to your partner's complaints to determine their love language on how you can better love them. Take Dr. Gary Chapman's quiz at 5lovelanguages.com. You can also find more on his teachings in his books or radio shows. Learning each other and taking care of your "teammate's'" needs takes decades if not until death do you part. Don't criticize your spouse in front of your children and others. Be a committed fan of your spouse, and brag about the person you love!

Remarried and blessed in a second relationship.

Is your ex remarried or happy in his/her next relationship? Or are you remarried, blessed and happier now? Why? Because they submitted or you submitted, learning from past relationship mistakes. You or your ex now know what it takes to make marriage successful. The things he or she/you ran from, the things your partner and you needed to overcome in the first marriage, he or she/you did in the second marriage. I ran in my first marriage. Now I know better and I have the tools to do better thanks to my marital counselor, Glory. Are you still running? Or are you fighting and doing what it takes to make it work? To be great at anything you have to put in thousands of hours, and this includes relationships. Instead of running from your problems, solve it with God and find peace in your heart.

Are you just roommates with living arrangements?

That's not good for anyone. LL4 and I were definitely roommates as were my parents. It takes courage for either party to see this and for both to be willing to work on the marriage and relationship at the same time. Get over the hurdle of your own hurt. Love your partner so you can change the climate of your relationship. There is far more potential in reaching out in loving someone versus condemning them.

You can't have a good marriage unless you discuss the things that annoy you first.

If you can't build a foundation with healthy communication and solve problems you encounter before marriage, then you shouldn't be married. Furthermore, if you come off the high of being in a relationship, it's because you haven't built a foundation.

"It's much easier to turn friendship into love then love into friendship." - *@AverageBlackMan on Twitter*

Consider how hard it is to change yourself and you'll understand what little chance you have in trying to change others.

Patterns from childhood often recur in adult relationships unless essential efforts are made to change. The best thing in life is finding someone who knows all your mistakes and weaknesses and still thinks you're completely amazing! We are all messed up in our own special way. Don't look for a lover to solve your problems, just find one that doesn't let you face them alone.

Work together as a couple and individually on your relationship with God.

He created marriage and He is the one to turn to both individually and as a couple to make it work and to strengthen your bond. Don't let other priorities get in the way.

"As I've journeyed through life, one lesson I've learned is that every person in my life who has inspired me has gone through some sort of life altering event. Think about that for a minute and I challenge you to find someone who has not. Ghandi, Martin Luther King, Jr., Abraham Lincoln, Oprah, Joseph in the Bible, the list goes on. The reality is that as harsh as it may seem at the time, without that hardship to mold and transform you, you would not have grown as greatly as you did in the end. Their stories have a common thread. One of humbleness, perseverance, a will to succeed, and hope." - Unknown

"The loneliest people are the kindest. The saddest people smile the brightest. The most damaged people are the wisest. All because they do not wish to see anyone else to suffer the way they do." - Anonymous

"You are responsible for your life. You can't keep blaming somebody else for your dysfunction. Life is really about moving on." - Oprah Winfrey

"No one lives long enough to learn everything. They need to learn starting from scratch. To be successful, we absolutely, positively have to find people who have already paid the price to learn things that we need to learn to achieve our goals." - Brian Tracy

Strength is nothing more than how well you hide the pain. - Unknown

As much as you want to plan your life, it has a way of surprising you with unexpected things that will make you happier than you originally planned. That's called God's will. He will give you all you desire only after He transforms your character and aligns your heart with His. - Derived from Psalm 34:7

Learning comes with ups and downs. Often, learning is not fun but that's how we get to the next level in any aspect of life. If I'm always successful, am I really doing anything meaningful? I've failed several times in my life at all sorts of things and I am perfectly OK with that. God picks people for certain things; be happy for what you have and what you don't. Becoming a wife, a husband, a mother or a father doesn't just happen. You grow into it and work your ass off! I am definitely looking forward to the next chapter of my life: motherhood!

Thank you for reading my book.

Other Titles Available From

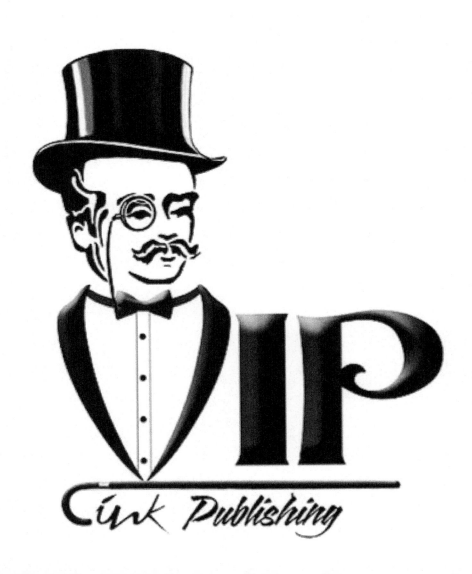

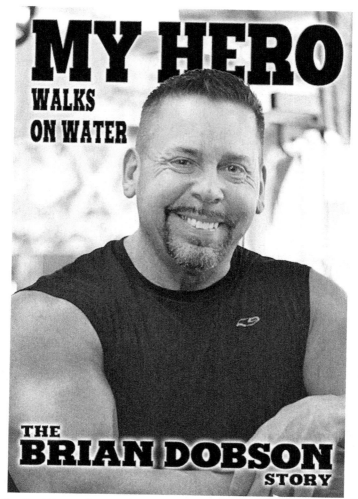

MY HERO
WALKS ON WATER

THE BRIAN DOBSON STORY

My Hero Walks On Water details Brian Dobson's amazing life story from the numerous times God has him to save people, when they felt they had nowhere else to turn, his discovery of eight time Mr. Olympia Ronnie Coleman. Dobson, founder of Metroflex Gym, is also trainer and mentor to Branch Warren, two time winner of the Arnold Classic Championship, and IFBB Pro Body Builder Cory Matthews. Metroflex gym is not your average gym. At times, it has been used as a ministry to help many people overcome addictions and to witness to them the message of Jesus Christ. In 2008, Dobson started a homeless outreach ministry that feeds over 500 people each month. The meals are provided with fresh meat and fish that Dobson personally catches. Dobson's philosophy is "this is exactly what Jesus would do". Forward written by eight time Mr. Olympia Ronnie Coleman. Contributors to the book include: two time winner of the Arnold Classic Championships Branch Warren, World's Strongest Bodybuilder Johnny O. Jackson, and Pastor Troy Brewer.

ISBN 13: 978-1939670083

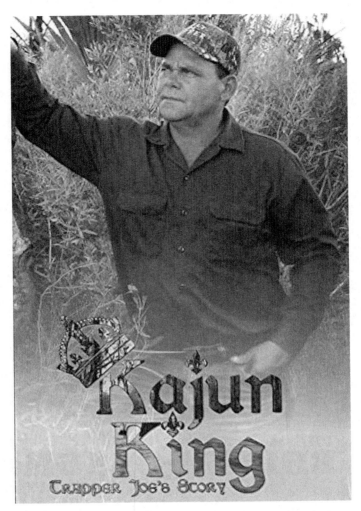

Kajun King

Trapper Joe's Story

Noces Joseph LaFont, Jr. (Trapper Joe) is a veteran when it comes to south Louisiana hunting and fishing. His traditional Cajun roots implanted in him as a child have been showcased on the hit television show Swamp People that airs on the History Channel. Alligator Season is the most exciting time of the year for alligator hunters in Louisiana. When Trapper Joe is not hunting alligators, he is hunting for other game within the Cajun lifestyle such as: fish, crawfish, shrimp, crabs, raccoons, turtles, deer, hog, rabbit, dove , and so forth. His autobiography details his life from growing up in the south Louisiana to helping Swamp People become the #1 rated reality show on the History Channel with a premiere viewing of 3.1 million. It is filled with amazing hunting and fishing stories as well as his Cajun recipes. This book is a real must have for any true fan of the Cajun lifestyle.

ISBN 13: 978-1939670236

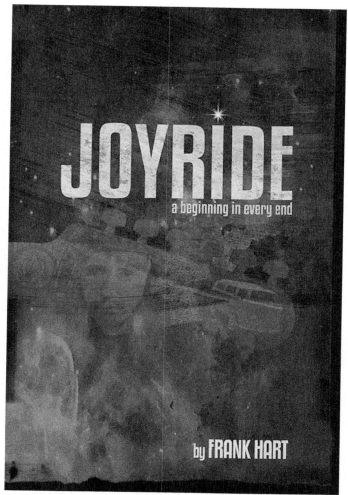

JOYRIDE
a beginning in every end

by FRANK HART

There are a lot of reasons why you might read a book. Maybe you want to be entertained, maybe you want to be inspired, maybe you want to peek into the secret closets and junk drawers of an almost famous, almost rock stars psychology. This is the story of a Mid western son of a coal miner who couldn't decide between a pulpit and an electric guitar. If you are interested, I'll tell you how I saw God in my backyard while Looking up at the stars and I'll tell you about coming so close to my wildest dreams that I could have licked the frosting with my tongue. Joyride was supposed to be the song that put my band, Atomic Opera, on the map. What? you have heard of Joyride? Exactly. You know the difference between a happy ending and a tragedy? It's all where you stop telling the story. -Frank Hart (Front man for Atomic Opera, a hard rock band from Texas that , along with King X's and the Galactic Cowboys, was part of Wild Silas Music works. The band was signed to Warner Brothers Records, released four albums and toured with Dio. Frank is now a worship leader and preacher and New Church in Katy, Texas, he has released two solo albums and continues to rewrite the ending of his story.)

ISBN 13: 978-1939670229

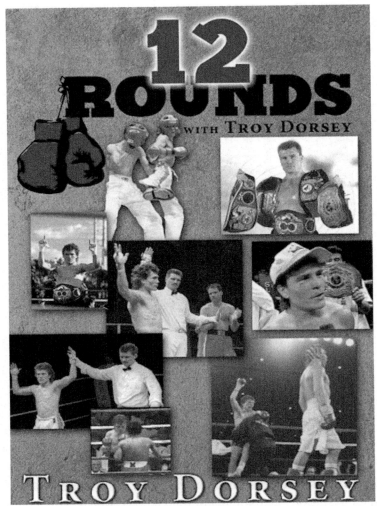

12 ROUNDS
WITH TROY DORSEY

TROY DORSEY

Eight time World Boxing and Kick Boxing Champion Troy Dorsey tells all in his book 12 Rounds. Troy Dorsey is a former professional boxer and martial arts fighter. As well as the first man in history to hold world titles in both karate and boxing. After a brief and successful run as an amateur kick boxer, Dorsey turned professional. He won multiple International and World Kickboxing titles sanctioned by K.I.C.K., ISKA, and Wako. Milestones of Dorsey's Kickboxing career include: a one sided knockout defeat of highly regarded Santae Wilson for the US Featherweight Championship and his literal destruction of a #1 challenger Steve Demechuk. Dorsey would drop Demechuk no less than 6 times before finally knocking his opponent out. Dorsey is widely considered one of full contact kickboxing's greatest fighters and a much sought after trainer. In 1985 Dorsey became a professional boxer. As a boxer, Dorsey held the NABF Featherweight Title, IBO Super featherweight Title and also won IBF Featherweight World Championship. His style and endurance made him one of the era's most exciting fighters. Troy Dorsey is perhaps best known for two non-stop fights with IBF World Champion Jorge Pàez in Dorsey's first title attempt. Milestones in Dorsey's boxing career include: brutal battles with Champions Gabriel Ruelas, Manuel Medina, Kevin Kelly, Jesse James Leija, and Tom Johnson, as well as, facing Olympian and future 5 time World Champion Oscar De la Hoya. With feature contributions by: World Champion Gene "Mad Dog" Hatcher, 2x World Champion Jesse James Leija, World Champion Stevie Cruz, UFC World Champion Guy Mezger, World Champion Paulie Ayala, and Hollywood Super Starr Bob Wall to name a few.

ISBN 13: 978-1939670106

CPSIA information can be obtained
at www.ICGtesting.com
Printed in the USA
LVOW04s1838160616

492905LV00016B/767/P